Praise for *Women's*

'Her advice is simple, friendly and explicit and ...
wonders.'
DAILY MIRROR

'A sizzling book.'
SUNDAY WORLD

'A sex manual which makes Jackie Collins' novels look tame.'
DAILY RECORD

'The nicest sex book I have ever read.'
SUNDAY EXPRESS

'Her frankness and humour make the discussion compelling.'
NEW ZEALAND DOCTOR

'Her central theme of regaining control over one's sexuality
goes to the core of why some women can't climax . . . a lot
of clean fun.'
THE WEEKLY JOURNAL

'Provides practical, common-sense answers to the serious
problems that many women (and men) worry about.'
HAMPSTEAD AND HIGHGATE PRESS

'As amusing as it is helpful . . . a wonderful understanding
of the baggage women bring to bed.'
NEW WOMAN (Australia)

RACHEL SWIFT

Fabulous Figures

or

HOW
TO BE
UTTERLY
UNIQUELY
GORGEOUS

PAN

First published 1995 by Pan Books Ltd

an imprint of Macmillan General Books
Cavaye Place London SW10 9PG
and Basingstoke

Associated companies throughout the world

ISBN 0 330 33543 X

1 3 5 7 9 8 6 4 2

A CIP catalogue record for this book is available from
the British Library

Phototypeset by Intype, London
Printed and bound in Great Britain by
Mackays of Chatham plc, Chatham, Kent

This book is dedicated with thanks to all the many women and men who wrote such wonderful letters of support for *Women's Pleasure*.

CONTENTS

ACKNOWLEDGEMENTS

The author and publisher wish to thank the following who have kindly given permission for the use of copyright materials.

Cambridge University Press for extracts from Ann Leader's 'The Association of Slimming with Eating Disorders', which appeared in *Proceedings of the Nutrition Society*.

Elsevier Science Publishing Co., Inc. for the graph on page 77.

HarperCollins Publishers for extracts from Shelley Bovey's *The Forbidden Body: Being Fat is not a Sin*.

IPC Magazines Ltd. for extracts from 'We've Had Plastic Surgery' which appeared in *Woman*.

John Wiley & Sons Inc. for the graph on page 12.

Macmillan Magazines Ltd. for extracts from Seilichiro Tarui's 'Visceral Fat Obesity: Anthropological and Pathophysiological Aspects', which appeared in *International Journal of Obesity*.

Jill Neimark for extracts from 'Slaves of the Scalpel' which appeared originally in *Mademoiselle*.

Random House UK Ltd for extracts from Judith Wills' *Size 12 in 21 Days* and Naomi Wolf's *The Beauty Myth*.

Routledge for extracts from Jane Ogden's *Fat Chance!*

She for extracts from Will Self's article 'The Erotic Charge of Large Women'.

W. B. Saunders & Co. for extracts from Kelly Brownell's 'Expert Opinion: Dieter's Weight Regained: Are There Risks?' which appeared in *Krause's Food, Nutrition and Diet Therapy*.

I would especially like to thank Catherine Hurley, my editor at Pan, for her patient and most helpful involvement with this book.

Every effort has been made to trace all the copyright holders but if any has been inadvertently overlooked, the author and publisher will be pleased to make the necessary arrangement at the first opportunity.

Why Is This Book Remarkable?

This is a book about what dieting is *really* like: which diets work and which ones kill you, what men really think about our figures, what the latest medical advances are, and what individual dieters have been through. It's full of facts and figures, attitudes, advice and funny stories.

It is also a celebration of real women – their uniqueness and their great variety. It is written for every one of the 90 per cent of women who diet, from the very largest down to those who are fading away from malnutrition yet who look in the mirror and see a 'fat' person. This book is about *all* shapes, all figures, *all women*.

Part One, (First, Choose Your Figure) is designed to help *you*, and not the faceless slimming industry, determine what is your ideal figure. You may be surprised to learn that the great majority of men do not demand a skinny partner, and indeed deplore women's constant attempts to diet. Rather than enhancing relationships, dieting frequently destroys them. The truth about dieting and health is equally surprising. I will expose the scandalous facts about height–weight charts, and produce remarkable new medical evidence, based on studies involving millions of people, to show that weight *protects* against disease, delays ageing, and increases fertility and sexual desire. Dieting, on the other hand, is positively bad for you: the case against it is getting more and more grim.

Part Two (What Are the Options for Losing Weight?) presents a sixty-page review of the notable slimming techniques and diet books, from the bizarre, via the familiar, to the downright dangerous. I review the surgical options for weight loss, and also reveal how the current obsession with dieting is blighting our children's lives: girls and boys as young as nine are suffering from anorexia, and eating disorders are on the rise the world over.

In Part Three (What Really Works?), for those of you who still feel you need to lose weight I shall explain in the form of a simple plan how to succeed permanently and safely.

Why Do We Suffer So?

Thirty-five years ago fashion models weighed about 10 per cent less than the weights recommended on the weight charts. Today, they are up to 19 per cent below their expected weights.

Think about that.

Over the last ten years, however, the weight of models and beauty contestants has remained more or less constant. Why? Because our role models have now become so thin that they satisfy one of the main diagnostic criteria for anorexia nervosa, namely, being more than 16 per cent below their recommended weights. It is now physically impossible for them to get any thinner without being holed up in an anorexia clinic.

The current ideal of ultra-skinniness that is thrust at women a thousand times a day – in magazines, films, television, books, advertising and doctors' surgeries – is very recent indeed. The other day, browsing in a second-hand bookshop, I picked up a delightful volume entitled *The Art of Beauty* by 'A Toilet Specialist', published at the turn of the century. The author, whom I shall be quoting throughout this book, enthuses about the 'plumpness which is one of women's charms', and sympathizes with 'the distress which want of adipose tissue may cause' . . . 'for it is natural enough that the woman should sigh for more ample proportions'.

As recently as the 1950s the fashionable female figure was very much more voluptuous than it is today.

It is not only a question of time, but of culture. Today, 80 per cent of the world's cultures consider plumpness desirable in women, 90 per cent of cultures consider large hips and thighs attractive. Yet women in the West, instead of celebrating their diversity and beauty, spend hours each day criticizing their bodies and semi-starving themselves. Many now pay surgeons to *cut* them into shape.

Who benefits from this madness? Well, the dieting industry does, to the tune of some £26 billion a year in Britain alone. Oh yes, and the plastic surgeons. But that's about it.

As for the rest of us? Wives, tired, cross and depressed from going without food, bicker with their husbands. Women of every shape and size feel uncomfortable with their bodies, are perpetually trying to change them, become obsessive about food and get fatter because of it. Women in a whole range of professions – dancers, actresses, air hostesses, receptionists, even shop assistants – wage a constant battle to eat less than they want because gaining a few pounds means losing their job. My friend Nerys, a hairdresser on a cruise ship, had a perfect figure, well within her ideal weight range, but was told she must lose 10lb or risk the sack. In this way the madness spreads, because the women whose hair she dresses will now feel fat by comparison. School children refuse lunch and perform badly in class. A whole new generation – male and female – is growing up with potentially lethal eating disorders. Even supermodels would be happier if they could spend a little more of their millions on food!

I asked a handful of women what they considered an ideal figure. Their answers were all along the same lines:

Thin, very very thin.

No horrible hips or bottom.

A boyish look – lean and sinewy.

A wonderful figure? Anything that's two stone less than I am.

But men have different ideas about women's figures:

Curvy – going in and out in the right places.

Something to get hold of – not all skin and bone.

For God's sake, something different from a man's figure!

What constitutes a gorgeous figure? All of them! The lot – the great variety, from the thinnest to the fattest.

And what did they think of Marilyn Monroe? Fat, fat, fat, said the women. Swoon, swoon, swoon, said the men.

The real tragedy is that never before in history have women had so much to offer, and so many opportunities to promote themselves as individuals and equals. And yet, never before has fashion been so uncompromisingly rigid about the way the desirable female body should be.

We need *energy* for our work – and that means eating properly.

We need *time* to train for new careers, to study and travel – and that means not wasting hours poring over boring diet books, weighing and measuring each ounce of food.

We need *money* to take advantage of our leisure – and that means not squandering it on diet pills, potions and products that we know in our heart of hearts won't work.

We need *self-confidence* to win top jobs and organize our lives – and that means not looking in the mirror and seeing our beautiful bodies as worthless and 'disgusting'.

It has taken me two decades to realize that dieting not only makes you fat, it also makes you cross and anxious, snappy, grouchy, miserable, depressed; it wastes hours and days and weeks and years of your precious life and sometimes it kills you.

It has taken me most of my life to accept that by finally stopping dieting, by throwing the bathroom scales out of the window, by lighting the fire with my calorie-counting books, not only am I reclaiming massive parts of my life, allowing myself to have a happy and carefree attitude to one of the greatest pleasures – eating – but for the first time in years *I am losing weight*.

I can hardly remember a time when I wasn't in some way anxious about being too large. Yet I was a rather skinny child. Where on earth could such ideas have come from? Partly, of course, from the fashion world. Yet it would be too simple to leave it at that. Delightful woman though she must have been, I also blame my great-grandmother, Alice.

Alice Miles, a true Victorian spirit (with plenty of crankiness thrown in), was a fervent believer that children should be never heard, seldom seen and only rarely fed. Perhaps she was disgusted by the gross indulgence that she saw around her when she was a young woman in the 1870s and 1880s – the seven-course dinners, the breakfast tables groaning with kedgeree, kidneys, scrambled eggs, chops and cold meats. Whatever the reason, Alice had a perfect mania; everybody ate too much, especially children.

This was inconvenient for her husband Herbert. Not only was

he a tall strapping chap who rather enjoyed his food, but he was also the Quartermaster General, in charge of the eating arrangements of the entire British army. With a job like that it seemed a particularly harsh injustice that he should be denied food at home. Their otherwise happy marriage echoed with constant arguments about what they ate, with Alice, if ever his concentration was distracted for a moment, leaning over and quietly removing potatoes from his plate.

I never knew Alice or the QMG, but Alice's influence persisted. Their daughter Gladys, my grandmother, in whose company I spent much of my childhood, was half-starved in her youth and never thereafter acquired a proper appetite. I've known her to get halfway through a boiled egg and stop, too full to continue. She had a curious habit of cutting food in half. At tea, she'd reach out, cut herself a slice of cake, cut this in half and eat the half. Later she might cut the half in half and eat that, and later halve the quarter.

Extreme slenderness suited her perfectly. She grew up as tall and willowy as any catwalk model today. By the time I knew her well she was approaching ninety, and as elegant as ever – more so, I suspect, for she had somehow accumulated nine decades of style and, as she never threw anything away, nine decades of elegant clothing. I once accompanied her to a party, at which she wore a black taffeta circular skirt from the 1950s, complete with wide stretchy belt, a blue and white polka-dotted 1930s crepe blouse, and a black velvet wide-brimmed Edwardian hat. With a role model like that, was it any wonder that I felt ungainly by comparison?

My whole family was skinny. Obviously, God intended me to be a skinny, too. But at my christening there was an omen: my grandmother, who leaned over my cradle, took one look at me and exclaimed: 'Goodness me, she looks just like my father, the Quartermaster General!' It seems that sturdy trencherman was going to shape my destiny.

My mother is not only thin but one of those oddities of nature who actually prefer an apple to a bar of chocolate. She had admirable, rather advanced views on nourishment for babies and went to great efforts to squeeze quantities of carrot juice for me to drink. I grew into a healthy, strapping teenager – and blamed the carrot juice. Why did my mother have to set me up so sturdily? Why couldn't I have been one of those peaky children with a 'poor start in life'?

By the age of fifteen I was well on the dieting road: at 5 ft 9 ins and 11 st, I felt enormous, though such a weight is well within the recommended range. But it sounded awful. 'I mean, that's what boxers weigh,' I wailed.

Ironically, while I was wailing, three friends at school were turning anorexic, wasting away in a misery ten times more serious than mine. I'd scarcely heard of the disease then. What mystified me was that all three girls were already skinny – why on earth should they want to diet?

In my late teens I enjoyed a year or two of thinness before I took the Pill, and that was the beginning of it all again. The battle had begun in earnest – a battle which, I don't doubt for one moment, would never have been necessary if I had not begun dieting. Had I simply accepted myself the way I was instead of trying to be Twiggy, I would have stabilized around 10 stone, a delicious, slightly curvy shape. Instead, my life has been that of the average dieter – a steady sequence of starving, scoffing, lazy indulgence, defiant eating, ashamed dressing in black tracksuits and, once again, resolute dieting. I remember in my twenties thinking that there was hardly an hour of my waking life that passed in which I didn't in some way feel too fat. A stray chance comment such as 'size 14, madam?' – a size I now see as ideal for my height – would haunt me for months. For life is perhaps a better description, as many of these remarks I shall never forget; and though they would not sting me now, the sting they gave then does not diminish. If that sounds bizarre let me add that since researching this book I realize that my own obsessions were relatively mild by comparison with many women's.

When people told me I was not fat, I knew they were saying it just to appease me. Sometimes, in exasperation, friends would remark, 'For goodness sake, you're large, big build, not fat.' But that comment was the most appalling insult of all. Fat at least could be got rid of, but *big build* – to me it conjured up visions not of a statuesque Princess Michael whose strong bold looks will remain long after the skinnies have shrivelled away, but of a lumbering zombie.

In pursuit of fashionable flat-chestedness I went through a phase of walking everywhere clutching a large book to hide my bosom. My friend Fanny's trick was to take up smoking; between drags she kept her right arm, cigarette in hand, pressed stylishly against her chest, smoke getting in her eyes, like fashionable women of the old Hollywood movies. Now I see women enduring pain and real danger to obtain, through surgical breast implants, what we were constantly trying to obscure. It breaks my heart to think of the wasted hours and years I spent in misery over something which I now know to be an asset.

Like most young women, I was concerned about male approval, yet when boyfriends told me not to diet I thought they were mad. The fact that I never had any trouble finding them in the first place, or drawing appreciative glances in the street, did not register. Clearly that was in spite of my shape, not because of it.

At university I moved into a flat with my best friend Julia, also a compulsive dieter. Our efforts to lose weight reached new heights, but at least we could laugh about it. When I bought a pair of very trendy purple leather boots with zips from Chelsea Cobbler and found they were too tight to do up, we developed a useful technique: lie on your back, wave your legs in the air, insert a coat-hanger hook into the zip and pull. Then all you have to do is stagger to your feet and hobble off into the sunset. It works quite well on tight jeans too, if you don't mind going without air for an hour or two. I was constantly buying clothes a size too small 'because I'm about to lose 7 lbs'. Julia was more sensible: she had two wardrobes, one large and one small.

We went off on holiday to India together. At the airport we worried that, with the price of fuel, it was only a matter of time before airlines started giving each passenger a weight allowance which had to include the person as well as the baggage. Sorry visions arose of us queueing sheepishly with one minute holdall while all the skinny women could afford heaps of baggage.

In India it struck me that if I could only get a bout of dysentery, all my weight problems would be solved. So while Julia ate and drank cautiously, I swallowed unboiled water and suspect local market foods. Julia got the dysentery.

And so the endless weight-loss/weight-gain struggle continued.

How did I stop? Nothing dramatic, really. To a large extent it was a matter of confidence: being successful as a writer was the first step. Then something very obvious struck me: either do something about it and lose weight permanently, or stop worrying. It's crazy to do both. At long last I realized that life is no better when you're a sylph. After all those years I had actually got so accustomed to me as I am that the idea of becoming very thin was quite appalling.

I started listening to other people – my partner in particular – and believing what they said.

Most of all it was seeing the miseries that other women underwent in their despair over their shape – very often thin women. Looked at objectively it seemed absurd: why should I participate in that?

Gradually I stopped the constant preoccupation with weight. I began eating properly and exercising moderately. Gradually I have become less obsessed with food and my weight has stopped seesawing all over the place. It is going down slowly but surely to the weight that suits me best. If there were a magic pill to make me any size I liked, I'd choose $10^1/_2$–11 st – for someone of 5 ft 9 ins and my build that's a size 14 dress, and 30–32 ins jeans. Nothing would induce me to be thinner. Why? Because, clearly, I was never meant to be that thin: I would not recognize myself. A bit of substance keeps you healthy and youthful.

But this book will be nine months in the press – I'm quite sure readers will understand why it's wise to make no predictions about what size I end up then!

Join the Campaign!

This is also a campaigning book.

I started writing it because I was aware that thousands of women, like me, suffered agonies over dieting. What has astonished me is the staggering number of women – often beautiful, successful, strong, slim women – whose lives are disrupted by debilitating eating disorders and perpetual self-criticism. We women have put up with this truly horrible anxiety for far too long. Most of us know in our heart of hearts that dieting does not work, but we go on bashing away at it – because we feel weak if we give up, guilty that it must be our fault. Let me say once and for all: dieting has proved universally the most abominable way to lose weight!

My message is not that we should give up trying to lose weight. Clearly that is unrealistic. It is only that we need to re-evaluate what is an attractive size to be. If we can just slow the dieting madness down a bit we will see that gorgeous figures come in all sorts of sizes. We will see that the truth about health and weight is very different from what we have been led to believe, and that, except in very exceptional cases, dieting is making us all larger.

Five years ago such a book would have sunk like a stone. Now it is different. Courageous women all over the world are refusing to be intimidated into feeling they are worthless unless they are super-thin.

Together We Can Put a Stop to This Madness

So, do not think of this as a private book, an exchange between two people, me and you, author and reader. As you read, imagine the millions of women all over the world, many of them far more tightly caught in the dieting trap than you are, though they may look sleek and happy. And when you have finished reading, let's all have the courage to say 'Enough is enough'. There are happier ways to live our lives.

Part One

FIRST, CHOOSE YOUR FIGURE

1

Women's Greatest
Asset . . .

I see scarecrows
I see skeletons
I see no juicy pumpkin women

Korean poet on visiting England

Women's greatest asset is variety. We come in a glorious range
of shapes and sizes, and we have an almost infinite variety of
hair and clothes styles available to us. Yet we all – or several
million of us at least – apparently wish to look like Cindy Crawford,
Princess Diana or whoever the model of the moment is.

How dreary!

We'd save ourselves an awful lot of needless worry if we gave up
the attempt and simply revelled in the qualities that make each
one of us unique. We all strive for individual personalities, yet
when it comes to bodies we are all terrified of not conforming.

It has not always been this dismal. The histories of art, literature
and fashion are filled with more beautiful, various, shapely women
than even Father Christmas could deliver. So next time you are
feeling really unhappy about your shape, don't sit around moping,
or cook yourself a gigantic meal (you can do that later), or rush
out and join a dreary old slimming club. Instead, take yourself off
to your nearest art gallery, museum, public library or good bookshop and spend a pleasant half hour concentrating on history's
fabulous figures.

'It's all very well to look at them,' objected my friend Lorna,
'but what relevance can they have to me today?'

The relevance is this: looking at these women you will see that
we are today just one tiny part of a great, constantly changing

historical process. And we all have the power to hasten the change. Extreme thinness will not always be an ideal, any more than it has been in the past.

There is a further, more profound, point. When I began writing this book I thought it would be interesting to include a section on how ideas of beauty have varied over history. But a bit of research quickly showed that such a task was not only impossibly difficult but also insignificant. Out of the huge pool of human shapes and sizes, faces, figures and styles, fashion selects a particular type to grace with its attention, but this is an artificial choice. It no more represents what the people of the time consider the only truly desirable type of woman than a robin represents the only type of bird. Those voluptuous ladies of the eighteenth century were arrogantly called ideals, just as Cindy Crawford is today, but at neither time – thank heaven! – were the ideals of the general public so ridiculously narrow. In fact, it is more helpful to look at it the other way round. If you put together all the ideals that have ever been promoted during history, what you have is an indication of the range of female types and figures that are delighted in around the world every day. In short, if fashion has ever promoted your type of figure, then you can be sure that your type of figure is still admired today. And let me tell you right now, there are very few types that fashion has left alone.

Yet any woman under eighty-five years old might be forgiven for believing that a thin figure is a God-given ideal. After all, the 1920s was a decade of skinnies, wasn't it? All those boyish bobbed haircuts, flattened bosoms and straight tube dresses. And, with the brief exception of the 1950s when hips and bosoms reappeared, it's been much the same ever since, give or take an inch here and there, hasn't it?

Absolutely not. Even the 1920s was not in fact a decade of skinnies. Those Twenties flappers were the exception, not the rule. They have come to personify the decade because they were *new* – not *numerous*. They grabbed the headlines. As my super-sylph grandmother laughingly told me:

> Your idea of the Twenties is focused on a small minority, the so-called Bright Young Things who scandalized society. They're remembered, not least because novelists like Evelyn Waugh, Aldous Huxley and William Gerhardie wrote about them. A lot of people tried to copy them, and certainly

4

Twenties fashions looked more elegant on a boyish figure. But most women, emerging from Edwardian ideals of shapeliness, could not shed their flesh so conveniently, nor did they wish to!

For the minority, bent on being fashionable no matter what, 'the Roaring Twenties were,' writes Hillel Schwartz, 'the calculating, calorie-controlled, ounce-conscious Grim Twenties'.

I have the proof that figures were more various than we suppose upstairs in my own attic, in a collection not only of old snapshots but also of antique clothes. Among the latter, for every slinky, skinny, gold lamé creation there are three or four extremely ample dresses. Among the piles of photographs – which range from the 1880s right up to the 1960s – one sees every figure imaginable. What *has* changed in recent years – and it is an ominous development – is that almost all women (and children) now feel that they ought to be boyishly thin. Before, there was a much greater tolerance among women of a variety of shapes.

Ever since the fashion for extreme slenderness got going, most women have been having a struggle. Models today weigh less than 90 per cent of the population. Many of them are well over 20 per cent lighter than the average woman of their height. More than ever before, fashion's narrow conception of what a model must be is divorced from the enormous, rich variety that exists and the range of figures that are really admired, wondered at, respected and loved.

Let me give just a few examples to prove my point.

'Ideals' of the Past

In future, when aesthetic refinement will be more common . . . what an impetus will then be given to the development of Personal Beauty! Refined mouths and noses, rosy cheeks, sparkling eyes, plump and graceful healthy figures, now so lamentably rare, will then become as plentiful as blackberries in the autumn.

Henry Theophilus Finck,
Romantic Love and Personal Beauty, 1887

It is particularly satisfying that the very earliest women to gain modelling contracts, those in the Gravettian period of the last ice age, around 25,000 years ago, were absolutely enormous. Extremely accurate statues (known as Venus figurines, after the Roman goddess of sexual love) were carved of them. The star, the 'Venus of Willendorf', would, at a guess, have worn a size 30 sealskin dress and a 44GG bra. No one is quite sure who these women were. One suggestion is that they were the women in charge of the supply stores, and their size was a reflection of their beauty and prestige. Other experts have suggested they were examples of early pornography, and still others that they were fertility figures. In either case, big (very big) was beautiful (nowadays some measly little doctor would wire their jaws up).

In prehistory, losing weight happened by force of circumstance. Up until 5000 years ago people lived in small, food-foraging societies. There was no farming: if you wanted a meal you popped out with a spear and basket in the hope of finding a woolly mammoth for the main course and a handful of blackberries for dessert. Naturally, it was not a particularly reliable method of providing supper. And when you add to this the various ice ages, the droughts, the waves of pestilence, the loss of habitats and the migration of herds, it is not surprising that skinniness was something to be avoided at all costs. Size protects against famine and disease. If anything, there would have been diets to increase the figure, such as some communities still have today. Among the Elfik of Nigeria, for example, pubescent girls are put into special 'fattening huts' for up to two years in order to bring them to marriageable size. Only the richest members of the community can afford such a pampering for their daughter (who, poor girl, is also subjected to a three-tiered hairstyle and a brutal clitoridectomy). The plumping method of the Havasupai of the American Southwest, on the other hand, is quite different: if a girl is too thin, a fat woman stands on her.

The Arabian Nights provides numerous examples of very fleshy women who set the local princes' and kings' hearts alight. Some are almost mythically large, especially around the buttocks: the woman who opens the door to Prince Diamond in the 911th night could not come out further to greet him 'because her backside, dimpled with valleys, was so remarkable a benediction that she could not move easily without it trembling like curdled milk in a Badawi's porringer or quince jelly heaped on a plate perfumed with benzoin'. And in the 526th night a slave girl who has been

6

taken to the king has her beauties described, the highest praise being 'that blessing of Allah, her most desirable bum . . . it was so vast that the merchant had not been able to find a veil great enough to cover it'. Large bellies are also considered highly desirable:

> From time to time the breeze lifted the filmy chemise to her navel, showing her belly, which was as white as snow, with dimples in delicate places, each large enough to hold an ounce of powdered nutmeg.
>
> 206th night (Mather's translation)

These are extreme examples. What is important is that at some stage in history fashion has applauded them. And, if they were popular once you can be quite sure that they are still admired today. I'll give you just two examples. In 1986 the demand for substantial men and women was such that a special dating agency had to be set up. Two-thirds of the men who join Plump Partners are not themselves large, but have joined solely to find a good-sized woman. My second example concerns pornographic magazines. To the astonished stares of my local paper shop assistants I bought a huge pile of 'girly mags' – from the high-class *Playboy* and *Penthouse*, through those with Readers' Wives sections such as *Fiesta*, right down to the seedier varieties. And yes, *most* of the women in these are significantly larger (in all directions) than the model ideals thrown at women in women's magazines and the like. In fact, there are a number of publications which feature nothing but 'larger ladies' – and very substantial they are too.

For most of human history, plumpness has been fashionable, not least because it has been (correctly) associated with fertility, and considered an insurance of good pregnancy and lactation. Indeed some scientists today believe that the epidemic rise in infertility in the West is due, in part, to excessive dieting by women.

Famously, Rubens lovingly painted not only enormous women but their cellulite too (go on, off to the bookshop if you don't believe me). The massive, soft, voluptuous women inspired – among scores of others – the French Impressionist Renoir. And for those women whose troubles are in the other direction, try looking at the svelte sylphs of the painter Modigliani.

(It is occasionally pointed out by ill-natured people that just because a painter paints a large woman this does not mean he

7

fancies her too, or that she represents a norm or even an ideal. This is a feeble argument for several reasons. First, painters often painted their own wives or mistresses. Second, and this is certainly true in the Renaissance, painters often painted nudes for rich patrons who used them, in effect, as high-quality pornography. Third, the sheer quantity of fleshy women throughout the history of art suggests that if they were not the norm, or even ideals, then painters must over the centuries have been engaged in some perverse plot to con future generations. And fourth, you only have to speak to painters about their work to realize they paint what gives them pleasure.)

One of the pleasures of reading old travel accounts is the way in which the travellers, visiting for the first time Russia, Poland, China or Argentina, describe the women they encounter: 'Fresh-faced, round, of a most comely constitution as to make even the stoutest of English ladies appear frail.' In Malcolm Bradbury's contemporary novel *Rates of Exchange* the Eastern European writer Katya Princip says, referring to her stomach: 'Here we think a fatness there is just a little erotic.' When I first visited India, aged twenty-two, I was a stone and a half over my 'correct' weight. On trains, and even in the street, I was often asked politely by men 'How do you keep your lovely figure?', 'What is your secret?'

The English classics are full of approving references to shapely, curvaceous women. In Jane Austen's *Emma*, Harriet Smith 'was a very pretty girl, and her beauty happened to be of a sort which Emma particularly admired. She was short, plump and fair . . .'. Jane Fairfax, however, is 'between fat and thin, though a slight appearance of ill-health seemed to point out the likeliest evil of the two'. The stories of Sherlock Holmes make it abundantly clear what kind of shape was most admired in the 1880s and 1890s, as, for example, Dr Watson's comment about a lady client in 'The Veiled Lodger': 'Long years of inaction had coarsened the lines of her figure, but at some period it must have been beautiful, and was still full and voluptuous'. Dr Watson would be amused to see how in recent years the West has recognized that the 'miracle' drugs of the twentieth century can be fallible, and consequently many doctors are turning to old remedies for safe, effective cures. In the same way, doctors of today are only now beginning to heed what our ancestors knew by long slow observation: namely, that flesh protects against illness. This is particularly so in the case of the typical female pear shape that in recent years has, alas, suffered rather a battering at the hands of fashion. Seilichiro Tarui, a doctor at Osaka University Medical School, has this to say:

> As far as paintings of beautiful ladies are concerned, from Rubens' 'Las Tres Gracias' and Goya's 'La Maja Desnuda', through modern paintings of the surrealist or 'déformé' schools, to contemporary pictures by Botero illustrating a marked fat accumulation, there seems to be a wonderful, but possibly unconscious, agreement that the lower segments of the female body should be emphasized. The aesthetic principle thus appears to be coincidentally in accord with health requirements.
>
> The only exception I have seen is Michelangelo's painting of Adam and Eve in the Vatican in Rome. Eve's body seems android [apple-shaped] and Eve in 'Paradise Lost' was also painted extremely strangely; this could be the strangest woman's body ever painted.

Before the Twenties, 'thin' almost always suggested ill health, in particular the dreaded pneumonia and tuberculosis. And although old novels frequently praise a woman for her 'slenderness' or 'delicacy', this is a comparative term, and certainly more substantial than the supermodel skinniness that we mean by those words today. I always remember how, reading Charlotte Brontë's *Jane Eyre* at school, our English teacher would give vivid descriptions of Mr Rochester's attraction to the voluptuous Blanche Ingram. Jane herself, we were told, was not a good specimen of Victorian womanhood, being thin and small; indeed part of the pleasure of the story is her triumph against impossible odds.

Golden Lotus, the heroine of the Chinese erotic classic of the same name, had 'a white belly yielding and plump . . . Words fail to describe the charm of so beauteous a vision'. So beauteous, indeed, that she was a positive health risk. On seeing her, the souls of men would flutter away and die. The poet Verlaine, very crude, is crudest of all about the charms of a substantial behind – 'truly, the breasts' big sisters . . . Praise and glory to you, O holy breasts, O majestic ass' – and very down on skinniness in a woman, except in the case of Rita, because she intriguingly reminds him of a man, and Verlaine is partial to either sex. Another Frenchman, Théophile Gautier, describes his vision of a desirable woman in *Mademoiselle de Maupin*:

> As to her figure, she is rather plump than thin. I am some-
> thing of a Turk in this matter, and I should scarcely like to
> meet with a corner when I expected a circumference . . . a
> subject of Giorgione's wrought by Rubens.

But you don't have to resort to erotic literature to prove the point:
teaching English as a foreign language will do just as well. When
during several spells as a TEFL teacher, I used to set my students
essays on the traits of their home country, invariably sex and beauty
would creep in. I found it almost a rule that the further east you
go, the more curvaceous women are admired. I have a postcard,
sent to me from Greece, of a belly dancer so magnificent she
makes Jayne Mansfield look feeble. Though she would certainly
be dismissed as 'fat' by slimming magazines, she always receives
admiring gasps from male visitors. And as for the ancient
Greeks . . . their models, be they young gods or sturdily curvaceous
women, have held their fascination for two thousand years. The
famous Venus of Praxiteles, unequivocally plump, was so provocative that one pilgrim to her sanctuary leaped upon her, and then
demanded that the sacristan open up the back of the shrine so
that he could see her from all sides.

Ancient Greece also provides one of the few examples of skinnies as an ideal, in the Cycladic dolls. These little marble statuettes
represent a sort of prehistoric flapper – a model with slight hips
and precious little in the way of breasts, whose femininity has been
minimized and who would not have looked out of style in the
Twenties and Sixties.

The concern with *weight*, rather than *shape*, is very recent. The
idea of weighing yourself began in the sixteenth century with an
Italian called Santorio. He was not interested in losing weight, but
in plotting the variations of it, and determining how the body
changed over time. For thirty years he measured everything; and
I mean, everything. ''Tis no unseemly thing to weigh the excre-
ment,' he announced haughtily, and then sat in his special weighing chair that was suspended from the rafters next to the dining
table.

In the middle of the eighteenth century, around the time that
George III was losing our favourite colony, America, there began a
European vogue for weighing oneself at shops, with large hanging
scales. (How unselfconscious they were! Have you ever seen any
woman step boldly on to that dreaded device, the I Speak Your

Weight machine? Surely it was invented for men and luggage only.) The Earl of Salisbury stood at 15 st 9 lbs (219 lbs) and when he came back eleven years later he was up to 19 st 4 lbs (276 lbs). The Bristol dandy Beau Brummell weighed himself more than forty times. Gross indulgence! Did he, I wonder, daintily remove his exquisitely fashioned shoes beforehand? In those days weight was *not* the sensitive issue it has become, as witnessed by a diary entry by Lord Molesworth, the man who first imported monkey puzzle trees into England, about a pleasant day spent with his wife which culminated in: 'Weighed Lady Molesworth.' Can you imagine a woman today letting her husband, as a loving gesture, lift her on the scales?

It wasn't until the second half of the nineteenth century that the first diet book appeared. William Banting, born in 1797, was a fashionable London undertaker of St James's Street. His life prior to the diet has the quality of a nightmare. Coming from a family which had no tendency to corpulence, he had, nevertheless, from childhood 'an inexpressible dread of such a calamity', and to his dismay discovered it creeping up on him in his thirties. Soon he could not tie his shoe, 'nor attend to the little offices humanity requires without considerable pain and difficulty'. He had to go downstairs backwards to lessen the strain on his joints, and, since 'moderate and light food was generally prescribed', his system was brought 'into a low and impoverished state, without decreasing corpulence'. The weight continued to accumulate and his eyesight became inhibited, and then he began to grow deaf. In August 1862, at the age of sixty-five, Banting was 5 ft 5 ins tall and weighed 14 st 6 lbs, 'a formidable weight for an elderly gentleman of sedentary habits'.

It was at this point that he consulted a Harley Street doctor who prescribed the diet that was to make Banting so famous and help him lose over three stone within a year. Banting published the diet, in a book entitled *Letter on Corpulence*: it was considered a publishing phenomenon because it sold 58,000 copies in four languages in fifteen years (compare that with the over 60 million diet books sold last year in the US alone). His name entered the English language and now appears in the Oxford English Dictionary defined as 'Treatment of obesity by abstinence from sugar, starch and fat'.

Banting died in 1878, by which time the drive for thinness had begun to gain a little momentum, particularly in America. But it

11

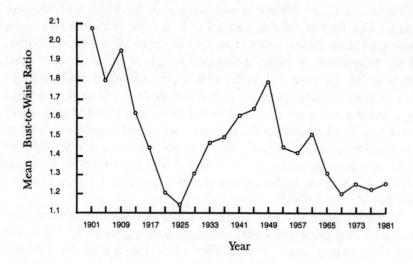

Figure 1

Mean bust-to-waist ratios of women appearing in *Vogue* at four-year intervals since 1901. (Taken with permission from Silverstein *et al.*, 'Possible Causes of the Thin Standard of Bodily Attractivensss for Women', *International Journal of Eating Disorders*, Vol. 5(5), 1986.)

was still more a question of how obese patients might lose their flab, rather than any overall drive for thinness: certainly nothing to be compared with the mania of nowadays.

In a delightfully earnest article published in 1986, five academics measured the busts and waists of thousands of photographs of women in copies of *Vogue*, dating from 1901 onwards. Plotting bust-to-waist ratio (which is not really so much a measure of slenderness as of curvaceousness) year by year, they recorded their results on a graph (see figure 1). By the 1920s, articles were appearing in the papers deploring the tendency of girls to starve themselves, and eating disorders became common. Even the American Bureau of Home Economics was worried, although for less than altruistic reasons: 'Economists have agreed that one of the outstanding reasons for the decrease of cereal consumption was the modish slender figure.' Great hope was put on the introduction of Empress Eugenie hats, first fashionable in 1931, which looked fetching only on a curvaceous wearer: anyone skinny looked a ninny. All around the country wheat manufacturers waited with bated breath to see if this would do the trick and force a 'drastic change in contour' among the nation's trendsetting females. And, as you can see from the graph, it must have worked, because the bust-to-waist ratio of *Vogue* models duly rose a little.

This female curvaceousness graph gave me the idea of doing a bit of research myself – instead of simply plotting 1901–82, why not cover the whole of history? After all, museums and art galleries are stuffed full of naked ladies from the last three thousand years. I duly set off with a tape measure to the British Museum, intending to calculate a relation between height and vital statistics. But I was doomed from the start, because old statues are often legless and decapitated – how can one measure accurately the height of a woman with neither legs nor head? Then again, some of the best statues are extremely tall, with quite inaccessible bosoms. And I had not reckoned on the museum keeper who, seeing me whisking out a tape measure and encircling every stone bottom in sight, evidently thought he'd stumbled on some very novel sort of pervert. So the ground-breaking Swift Female Ratios were not to be.

How Did the Modern Fashion for Skinniness Arrive?

Theories abound. Some people believe that the abundance and plenty of the West has led to feelings of guilt, and therefore punishment, fostered by Christian notions of denial as a virtue. Ann Hollander suggests that the shift from portraiture to moving images is behind it, because thinness is suggestive of motion and speed. Others have pointed out that figure shapes begin with *haute couture* and suggested that because so many fashion designers are homosexual men, the ideal has become as boyish as possible.

One fact often noted is that both the Twenties and Sixties represented periods of comparative economic power for women. Released from the confines of the home, where for centuries her primary function was child rearing, the new, professional woman (the theory goes) had to look different from the old housebound one. She had, in fact, to look more masculine. It's certainly true that people still have difficulty taking obviously feminine women seriously in the workplace. A test using computer-altered photographs showed that the same woman who, when flat-chested, was regarded as efficient and authoritative, when seen with a large bosom was no longer taken seriously. In my twenties I had long blonde hair, lots of curves (I still have those), and worked for a firm of architects. When I left, they gave me as a present black stockings and a suspender belt, along with the injunction that I must be sure to furnish the office with a photograph of myself wearing them. How can a person thought of in this way possibly be taken seriously? Suppose I had been given a managerial post? Would a woman feel respect for a managing director who posed for her in a black satin jock strap? So I have great sympathy for women who feel that in order to cut a dash in the business world you have to diminish everything that's obviously feminine – hips and bosom, or hair. Even the simple physical annoyance of bumping your bottom or bosom against someone as you pass them in a crowded office or lift makes size an issue for women at work.

Some writers see the obsessive drive for ultra-skinniness as a sinister way of oppressing women, by not permitting them any physical space in which to exist and by heaping debilitating anxieties upon them. It is, alas, a persuasive argument. As we shall see in Part Two, it is the clever high achievers who are most likely to be struck with eating disorders.

One thing is certain; whatever the cause of the ultra-thin obsession, women are party to it. But, if it is a means of keeping women in their place, isn't it an even greater imperative that we don't give in to it and connive at our own or other women's misery? Therefore, let's *all* stop feeling we must occupy as little space as possible, must look as much like men as we can, must starve ourselves and hate our own bodies. If we are to do battle in a very competitive male world we need all the strength we can get.

Personally, I think the mania for ultra-skinniness has many causes, some weighty, some trivial. The sixties, following on the revolutionary sex research conducted by Kinsey in the 1950s and then later pursued by Masters and Johnson, also began what one writer has called 'the era of the explicit'. Not only did corsets go out, but foreign holidays, suntans and exposing your flesh as much as possible came in. And, just to make sure the truth about women's bodies was as obvious as possible, Women's Lib insisted on daily bra-burnings. Then there was the matter of foods. Until 1959 the diet-food business was small, but in that year the American company Mead Johnson began a classic nationwide advertising campaign for a diet formula called Metrecal that had previously been promoted only in medical journals. It was so well managed, and so persuasive, that by 1961 the product had made US$100 million in sales. This, too, played its part in initiating the trend for extreme slenderness.

Twiggy, that marvel of malnourishment (remember the bumper stickers: 'Forget Oxfam, Feed Twiggy'?), didn't even appear on the scene until the mid-Sixties, by which time the skinny craze had long since begun. Far from initiating the boyish look, Twiggy represented the climax of it. As early as 1954 Christian Dior had shocked the fashion world by using the first ultra-thin models of the sort we have become used to today, in a landmark fashion show in New York. Five years later the Metropolitan Life Insurance Company of New York published their beastly height–weight charts which were widely publicized. It was, perhaps, these more than anything else that ensured the success of the rapidly growing fashion for slimming, despite the fact that we now know their recommendations to be fundamentally flawed. They gave vital 'scientific' underpinning to it, since the weights they recommended as 'ideal' for health were very low. As a woman I met who works on a famous fashion magazine once observed:

You have to think of the critical moments in fashion, such as the Twenties and Sixties, as arising from a mess of differing opinions and ideas with a force that is hugely disproportionate to the support the new fashion actually has . . . There are all these conflicting opinions about what's fashionable. Someone says skinny, another says hourglass, a third says voluptuous, etc. But then a scientist pops up and says: 'Hey, guys, we've just discovered that it's not healthy to be fat and we're about to publish a huge report to support this.' Followed by a modelling agent who exclaims: 'Look here! we've found this gorgeous waif, how about setting a new trend?' Followed by a dress designer who cries: 'Wow! there's this new artificial fabric that looks ace on skinny girls.' Succeeded shortly after by the food manufacturer who googles about his revolutionary way of producing low-fat foods. Fashion thrives on coincidence. Any one of these four might be enough to sway the balance. But all these factors – as happened in the Sixties – will obviously gather together like a wave in support of skinniness and overwhelm the counter-currents in support of hourglass, plump, voluptuous, all of which have previously had their day and still have their supporters. OK, so it turns out that the scientist was wrong, that there are other gorgeous models twice as large as Twiggy, that the fabric is horrible on most women, and that the new food makes your tongue taste like it's been coated in gloop – that doesn't matter. The dam has been breached. From now on the move towards skinniness is unstoppable. Fashion isn't natural. That's part of the excitement of it. It's totally artificial.

In other words, the thinness craze is one big, out-of-control merry-go-round. If more brave people made a stand against it – if fashion editors featured both skinnies *and* curvies modelling clothes, or film producers cast heroines who had a bit of shape to them – it would make an immense difference to us all.

Let's Enjoy Our Diversity!

Whatever the reasons for the skinny fashion that began in comparatively modest ways four decades ago, one thing is absolutely certain: it is no more correct, natural or obvious than any other fashion in the past. The main difference is that today we are particularly strongly influenced because the extent of our communications – TV, films, radio, newspapers, magazines – is greater than ever before. The skinny flapper look was interrupted by the Great Depression that began in 1929. Unfortunately, the very skinny look of the Twiggy era is with us still: fashion has got stuck in a rut, not least because the dieting industry has so much to gain from it. There has never been, in the history of the human race, so great a consensus that a certain 'look' is the 'right' one, the only 'fashionable' thing to be. It is this debilitating uniformity into which our gloriously rich and varied species is running head-long, that we must stop, and that we *can* stop.

Some months ago I answered a knock on the front door to find the Japanese translator of *Women's Pleasure* standing on the doorstep. She was visiting England and had stopped by to introduce herself to me. Eventually we began talking about this book. To my dismay, she told me that Japanese women too are getting hooked on the skinny ideal that began in the West:

Japanese girls are naturally sturdy, stocky even, and it suits them. They look beautiful as they are, and the boys, too, love them like that. But are they happy? No. Gradually they are trying to become thin like Western women. They've learned to hate their natural shapes, and they are beginning to starve themselves into new ones.

In Part Two you will see that medical statistics show that eating disorders, so terribly common in Britain and the US, are now spreading across Europe, Russia, even as far as Japan and other industrialized nations. This too is largely because of the effectiveness of global communications – the fact that we can 'see' halfway across the world simply by switching on a television. But the closer contacts we have with other countries mean it is all the more important that we do not try to impose our own conformity on them. Races differ in their body types and needs. A supermodel figure may be a cinch for Masai tribeswomen but it can be a living hell for a West Indian and a day-to-day misery for a Japanese girl, or indeed an Englishwoman.

Fashion has been positively influenced by the 'global-ethnic' look in terms of fabrics and styles, but shape has remained rigidly defined. I have already mentioned that of all the cultures in the world today an astonishing 80 per cent consider plumpness a sign of beauty in women. Yet our culture in the West – being so very powerful – is imposing its nasty little definition on the world. 'Corporeal imperialism' you'd term it, I suppose.

The same applies within our own country: now that we are so very multicultural and multiracial it is vital that we all stop trying to conform to a rigid, uncompromising body stereotype.

But all is not quite lost. I went recently to the Notting Hill Carnival, that vibrant West Indian celebration in song and dance, and here I saw the first glorious open display of women not hiding behind their differences but proud of them: figures of every shape and description adorned, paraded, worn with pride. Lycra was the popular material, and there was definitely no covering themselves up with stripes going in the right direction, baggy drab garments and all the 'camouflage' nonsense. As one writer described it:

Women who aren't gym-toned, with their big bottoms, bulging thighs and heavy breasts . . . wear Lycra. There's a contest as to who has the most biggest breasts, the most biggest bottom. What might not have been perceived as a great body becomes a great body and is flaunted.

Kowdo Eshun in the *Independent*

17

First, Choose Your Figure

I have a friend who used to be a famous fashion photographer, taking pictures of half-starved models for trendy magazines. Now he has turned his back on all that and works in Brazil. His most recent photographs of the Rio Carnival show visions that are marvellously inspirational to any dieter in this country: large, brilliantly adorned women dancing with complete abandon, heedless of all the inhibited, flesh-pinching fashions with which we are so familiar.

Now *that* is the way to be!

2

What Do *Men* Think About Women's Figures?

I've worked in a newsagent's for ten years and watched men and women buying their papers. The women are always picking up magazines telling them how to get thin and sexy, and the men are always picking up the top-row magazines which show very fleshy women. I sometimes wish they'd get together and sort out the contradiction!

Mrs Browne, Cheshire

There's no getting away from it, one of the main incentives to diet comes from a desire to be more attractive to the opposite sex. Many women just assume that 'being thinner' will make them more sought after by men in general, and more passionately desired by the particular chap they have in mind. Take me, for example. For twenty years I was constantly on one sort of diet or another; my weight veered wildly over a range of three stone, from reasonably slim to good and solid. But, regardless of what I weighed, every time I got a new boyfriend my first response was to rush home and begin starving, 'to make him even keener' as I thought.

This was all very well for the first week or so; the weight would come off very easily to begin with, I'd feel virtuous, and it seemed like fun. After a couple of weeks I'd get sick of dieting, stop losing weight and start seriously worrying about my figure. The result of this was I felt less self-confident and more anxious. I'd get snappy when the boyfriend tucked into a big meal that I felt I oughtn't to share. I'd get more inhibited – especially in the bedroom, where I'd sidle into bed well covered up in some voluminous garment. And so on and so forth – the obsession with 'being thinner' actually got in the way of the relationship in a hundred small ways.

Then one day, not so very long ago, a very simple fact finally sank in, namely that no boyfriend I've had has ever suggested I lose weight. Even at my stoutest I did not have difficulty finding a nice bloke. In fact, several boyfriends have begged me not to diet. Mrs Browne, the newsagent whom I quoted at the start of this chapter, has made a profound statement. There is a world of difference in the way men see women's figures and the way women see women's figures. And in the majority of cases (not all, I grant you, but the majority) the situation is very much more cheerful than the women fear. The vast majority of men do not demand a woman who is pencil thin.

Thinking carefully, this is certainly the impression I have gained over many years talking to men – even though I never had the confidence actually to believe it. But for the purposes of this book I decided to get straight to the point and conduct a survey to find out. I contacted all the men I knew, stopped milkmen in the streets and postmen on their rounds. I asked friends' husbands, shopkeepers, charity collectors, window cleaners, old and young. I even asked my neighbour's three-year-old, Willy ('Cuddly, cuddly womens' was his response). Their answers were overwhelmingly, *'NO! We do not demand skinny women'*. About a third of the men had individual rigid preferences: for skinny, slim, voluptuous, plump, petite, average, or whatever. Two-thirds said what they appreciated about women was their great *VARIETY*.

Several things about my little survey (aside from an enormous phone bill – men on the subject of women are very talkative) were remarkable. The first has to do with language. To different men, 'slim' can signify anything between a size 8 and a size 16. 'Slim' and even 'thin', as adjectives, have become such standard terms in the descriptions of beautiful women that they have ceased to denote simply a body shape. 'Slim', in particular, has become synonymous with beauty, to the point where some blokes when describing an attractive woman automatically say 'slim', even when she's wearing baggy clothes that defy body judgement. Conversely, if in describing a woman you add the word 'plump' or 'large' it is immediately taken that she's unattractive, although, in fact, she's considered by all extremely attractive. Many men agreed with this, once it had been pointed out to them. Robert:

> When I say 'slim' I see a beautiful, thin woman. I can see a beautiful bigger woman, but then I'd just say she was a beautiful woman with this lovely body. I don't actually go for very thin women myself, but if I ever say 'slim', immediately there's a picture of a beautiful model or actress. It's a chain of association, I guess. If there were ads of beautiful bigger women all over the place no doubt when you said 'plump' or 'large' it would immediately bring to mind one of them and then things would change.

The practical example of this is as Miranda describes:

> The funny thing is that whenever you get a man to describe his idea of an attractive woman, the adjective 'slim' or 'thin' is bound to appear in there somewhere. But when the same man later tells me he's come across the woman of his dreams and brings her round, lo and behold she's not in the least bit slim. 'So, where's Miss Skinnypants?' I say when she's gone. 'Wasn't she your ideal?'
> 'Oh, yes,' he says, 'but Flossie's different.' Or he says, 'So? That was just an abstract idea. Flossie is reality and if she ever leaves me I'll shoot myself.'

What men particularly noticed in women was confidence and dash. Alan:

> So you might not, in general, like really thin or really fat women, but that doesn't mean that one or the other couldn't, just because she was confident and sassy, seduce you, just like that. Of course she could. Attractiveness, sexiness, or whatever you call it, is much more interesting than just a figure. It's an attitude. Have you seen Nigerian women in those wonderful bright patterned clothes they have? They're the sexiest things on earth. Very big, but so confident, so enticing.

In other words, one of the most important aspects of being attractive to others (male and female) is *how you evaluate yourself.* The biggest favour you can do yourself is to think yourself just lovely.

Novelist Will Self, whose work I had never cared for, really won my admiration recently for an excellent article in *She* magazine (May 1994) entitled 'The Erotic Charge of Large Women'.

> What I find particularly sensually exciting about big women is that they very often give the impression of being more in touch with their bodies. When I hear a woman announce that she is going on a diet, I often feel like saying (given that she's not dangerously overweight, which is seldom the case): 'Make sure that you don't discard the part of yourself that is really the most valuable'.

Men, Just Like Women, Like Variety

Men, just like women, admire an enormous range of physical types. There are men who go only for very thin women, men who go only for very large women, and (probably the majority) men who will go for any body type provided they like the woman's looks, conversation, intelligence, humour and all the rest of it. It's perfectly straightforward and obvious. The trouble is, we don't believe the obvious. When my boyfriends used to say they didn't want me to get thin, I assumed they must be either demented or outstandingly polite. Several men I spoke to commented wearily on just this point. It was impossible, they said, to convince their partner that they didn't like women to be all skin and bone. Witness Jim, a twenty-five-year-old who works for the city council:

> I remember when I married my first wife I kept telling her to put on weight. That was in the Seventies. I kept saying that she should eat more and she thought I was mad. But I know no end of men who feel just the same. I mean, if size is all you've got to go on, then you're far better off with too much than too little.

One expatriate wrote:

> Part of the pleasure of coming to Spain was that for the first time in my life I wasn't constantly waging a battle with my girlfriend of the moment to try and stop her losing weight every second of the day. The Spaniards take a much more healthy view of flesh.

Nick, a man who made the unlikely transition from the National Theatre to cut-green-bean production, told me that for years he'd been thinking of writing a play which would open in the following way:

> *It is evening. The husband is waiting for his wife to come home. It is her birthday and he has prepared a special meal for her. He is pacing the room nervously. The door opens and she rushes in. They embrace, obviously very much in love, then they sit down to eat at the candle-lit table.*

> She: Mmmm, lovely. But only a small portion for me, I've got to lose weight.

> He: Darling, please don't. I love you as you are.

> She: No, no, I'm horribly fat. Please take those potatoes off my plate.

> He: But I prefer you as you are. I really do.

> She: Peter, *PLEASE – TAKE – THOSE – POTATOES – OFF – MY – PLATE!*

> He: What is this? Are you trying to make yourself less attractive to me? Have you got a lover . . . ?

'There are,' says Nick, 'all sorts of possible ends to this scenario. She might pursue her diet regardless and the whole play descend into farce. Perhaps she gives in, only to wake up the next day crosser than ever. Or she persists, gets the weight off, making her breasts, which Peter had been particularly keen on, go small and limp, and *he* gets cross and they have a row. Or . . . or . . . or . . . It's the perfect subject matter, there are so many permutations. Everybody could relate to it.'

Another classic husband/wife scenario occurs as they are both dressing for a party. The floor is strewn with clothes.

> She: It's hopeless, absolutely hopeless. I've nothing to wear.

> He (*surprised*): Why not wear the red?

> She: God, no! It makes me look horribly fat!

> He (*sincerely*): But darling, you look lovely in it.

> She: My God, are you blind or something?

Whatever their attitude to their partner's figure, many men feel excluded by women's attempts to diet:

> It's partly the ritual of it. The little dieting secrets, the weighing out of food, the patient self-denial. Perhaps that sounds silly, but I really do feel *excluded*.

And, what dozens of men complained about:

> I can't understand it. I tell her I love her as she is and she *still* puts herself through hell to get thinner. Why?

> I love my wife the way she is. She insists on dieting. Of course I don't own her, but what I cannot understand is that she really suffers on those diets. I mean I'd understand it the other way round, if I wanted her thinner and she just kept on eating, because eating is a pleasure. But why does she make herself less attractive to me *and* suffer for it?

Those fairy-tale stories of the doting, helpful husband who supports his wife all the way until at last she succeeds in shedding umpteen pounds or even stones and everyone lives happily ever after – those are very rare indeed. Not because men are all unhelpful beasts, but because most men don't care about it nearly as much as their partners do. They would far rather have their wife cheerful and relaxed, instead of grouchy and snappy day after day, as one is on a diet.

Often, they don't even notice if you do succeed:

> My girlfriend gives me hell. She's been going on this diet on the quiet, pretending she's not really going on it and that she's eaten all she wants in the kitchen or something like that. Then in the summer she throws off her clothes and puts on a bikini. I don't notice anything different and she throws a wobbly. ('Why are you throwing a wobbly?' I asked and she said 'Wobbly, wobbly, I'm not wobbly!') I tell her that she always looks beautiful to me but she's really angry because she's lost a stone and a half and I didn't even notice.
>
> Vic

So what's the difference? A stone or two or three here and

there? A big woman's dead sexy because she's got a body, know what I mean? A thin woman's sexy because she looks hard to grab hold of. Me, I like them all shapes, as long as they like me.

Gerald

So, remember: without doubt *you* are the severest critic.

There is plenty of other evidence to convince us that there is life over nine stone, if only we would pay attention to it. Velda has a particular trick:

> When I'm feeling fat and unlovable, I think of all the really happy married people I know, and the unhappily married ones. Are the happy ones glamorous and thin? Definitely not.

In my experience there's a definite tendency for opposites to attract: as a tall woman I'm frequently plagued by men of five feet nothing, and when I had long blonde hair I seemed to be a magnet for dark men. But, most importantly, I've noticed that people inclined to stoutness themselves seem to go for slim partners, and vice versa. I've lost count of the skinny men who complain about women being too skinny – which suits me very well, as I couldn't imagine fancying any chap who wasn't a lean bean. In fact I can't be too harsh on those men who insist on a Twiggy, because I insist upon the male equivalent. And I have every sympathy with Genette's favourite fantasy:

> I'm let loose in a World War II prisoner of war camp filled with emaciated but indomitable Englishmen, who before they got there were perfectly at home in a Spitfire, and never complained about rationing.

Will Self confesses that his own frame is sufficiently meagre for him to 'hide quite tidily behind lamp posts and parking meters'.

But it's thin *women* we're concerned with here, and surveys of attractiveness and beauty (in so far as such things can be meaningful) confirm that, in fact, today's average model is significantly thinner than most men find attractive. Of course, they like the model because she's beautiful, but they'd like her even more if she put on a stone or two. 'Men don't "spin out fashionable

25

images",' writes Naomi Wolf. 'indeed, research keeps proving that they are warm to women's real shapes.' Even among those cultures where a thin standard prevails, such as Britain and America, research shows that men like women to be plumper than women want to be. The American scientist Dr Symons believes there is a universal male attraction to plump women, irrespective of the cultural ideal being applauded at any given time.

But the cultural pressures on men *are* very great, especially on young men. Women are generally more tolerant of unattractive men than vice versa, but this has a lot to do with economic and cultural status. As women achieve more status and power, they are getting far more choosy. After all, if you can earn for yourself why put up with just any man? But for the moment I think it's safe to say that men are more susceptible to peer pressure. Show a group of men a selection of photographs of women of varying sizes and they will say they go for the fashionable shapes. But show the same men a collection of photographs when they're alone, and you get very different results: then they're prepared to admit that the more rounded figures are just as attractive, sometimes even pre-ferred. Will Self writes:

> I am prepared to out myself and proclaim my enthusiasm for the big woman, something I haven't been able to do until fairly recently because my past includes the same shameful proclivities as most men's . . . When I was younger, I was badly afflicted by the collective obsession with skinniness. For many years I would only have relationships with women who were extremely thin. I now realize that I couldn't see these women for what they were – as much victims of sizeism as I was. I also felt threatened, as many men do, by the biological reality of women, by their capacity for change and their seemingly close alignment with nature.

Of course men (at least the lower quality men) do have an annoying habit of huddling together at parties and discussing what sort of women they prefer – but even then the names that crop up are not usually the ultra-thin supermodels, but averagely slim actresses with personalities: Goldie Hawn, Felicity Kendal, Michelle Pfeiffer, and so forth. Men huddling in groups discussing women in front of women are especially tiresome. I've found that an excellent antidote to this is to carry round with you a collection of photographs of good-looking naked blokes culled from the new women's sexy magazines. The women are always eager to point out their favourite and the men realize just how daunting such behaviour is.

One thing I've noticed all my adult life is this: men hate going out to dinner with women who are faddy eaters.

> All women imagine they have to eat like flies. They worry they'll seem gross otherwise. I can't say it often enough: it's horrible. Unsexy, affected, uptight.

> How can *you* enjoy your meal if the woman's picking at hers? Especially when you know it's a pose and she's secretly envying yours.

> Women must think men are daft if they're going to fancy you less or more because of what you eat.

Will Self declares:

> Frankly, I'm fed up to the gills with sitting down to eat with women who are denying their true figure. It makes me positively glow when a woman orders a good meal and tucks into it with gusto . . . the sight of a big woman enjoying her body, either eating or dancing, is far more arousing than watching some animated trouser press perambulating down a catwalk.

All the same, when my friend and I shared a flat we used to go to the most elaborate lengths to pretend we were too delicate to eat, and meals before going out were standard. Once I was asked out unexpectedly by a chap who had turned up unannounced. I was fainting from hunger (on a diet as usual), not having had time for a furtive pre-dinner snack, and this called for some quick thinking. Inspiration came: I suggested we go to a café where my friend worked. On a trip to the loo, I arranged for her to smuggle me some extra food. Looking back on it I cannot help thinking how puzzled this chap must have been faced with a strapping great girl who apparently lived on air. Of course my friend and I were young, but such behaviour is very common, especially among teenage girls. In a more severe form it can be the herald of serious eating disorders.

The myth that dieting will improve your romantic relationship is one you would do well to reject, not least because a new trend is developing for marriages to break up because one partner has gone from dieting on to anorexia or bulimia. Indeed, an article devoted to the subject appeared in the *Guardian* last year. Sue Bland, a matrimonial lawyer, commented:

> While bulimia, like alcoholism, is an illness and therefore cannot be considered, in itself, grounds for divorce, the unreasonable behaviour it occasions may be.
>
> 27 July 1993

This includes not only extreme mood swings, but evidence of bingeing and vomiting left all over the kitchen sink!

Indeed, extreme plumpness can be a great romantic attraction, as the founder of the dating agency Plump Partners, Sandy Millington, found out. The man who later became her fiancé travelled two hundred miles for a first meeting, only to decide that at 13 stone she was too thin and that he would have preferred her if she'd remained at the 19 stone she had once weighed. Some men I've spoken to think it's almost a contradiction in terms for a woman to have a body like some of today's models.

> What's my ideal? Plenty to hold on to, someone whose body won't collapse at the first sign of trouble.

> I want a woman who has curves and flesh. I want a woman who looks comfortable as well as feminine.

> I'd never go for a woman below a size 16. Never. I did once and it was just all wrong. I like a woman of substance.

Or, as Inspector Morse's faithful Sergeant Lewis commented: 'I like 'em a bit plump meself.' And the late, ever-charming Anthony Burgess:

> I once went to bed with a top model. It was like going to bed with a bicycle.
>
> Speaking on the Wogan show

Many men are particularly against women trying to get rid of their hips, thighs and bottom:

I can't understand it. My wife even reads her diet books at breakfast. I thought the man was supposed to read at breakfast. I say to her, 'But I like you with hips and thighs. I married you for them.' Nothing will stop her. She reads diet books from morning to night.

A woman's meant to have big hips. She's meant to have curves. If I didn't want a woman with hips I might as well go for a man. It would be far easier to make a catch!

It's what the Greeks were supposed to bring to their art, wasn't it? That saucy poise that revealed the delicious femininity – her big hips and ass, in other words. No wonder it was called the Golden Age.

Shere Hite's *Report on Male Sexuality* is full of quotations from men praising women's bottoms.

Ian, a political columnist on an East Anglian newspaper, art critic and budding film director (i.e. a bloke of many talents and much perception) remarked,

I dread the day, truly, I dread it, the day when somebody discovers a diet that works. Imagine if all women had the same body. How boring! I mean to say, how would you tell them apart?

Another category of man that I came across is that of the type who had always thought that a conventionally slim figure was his ideal, only to find after an encounter with a more fleshy female, that his tastes had changed:

I fell in love with Sheena in spite of her figure rather than because of it, I must admit. All my other girlfriends had been thin, and Sheena was – well – fat I would have called her. But she enchanted me, her personality, her confidence, and I fell for her. Quite honestly I find it hard to remember that I used to go out with skinnies, she's so warm, so inviting, so utterly *comfortable* in bed. And that is very very sexy.

R.J.

29

I quite seriously believe that if a lot of men gave larger women a try – if their pinhead egos would permit it – they'd get an incredibly pleasant surprise.

Stuart

In talking to men one thing quickly became obvious: namely that figure was less important than something almost indefinable:

What women never seem to understand is that almost every woman is amazing to a man. When men first start having relationships with women they find it incredible that they should be so lucky. That something so wonderful as a woman could want *them*. Many men never lose that feeling. It's always there, which is why it just doesn't make sense to assume one figure is more sexy than another. It's the woman who appeals, not just the body. If it were just the body, then blow-up dolls would sell in their billions. They're much less trouble to get into bed!

Jimmy, who said the above, agreed that Naomi Wolf (never one to let men lightly off the hook) puts it very well in *The Beauty Myth*. She points out that men are interested in femaleness and its sexuality, rather than 'femininity', which she calls 'a code for femaleness plus whatever a society happens to be selling'.

In that sexuality, women are physically beautiful already; superb; breathtaking.

Many, many men see it this way too. A man who wants to define himself as a real lover of women admires what shows of her past on a woman's face, before she ever saw him, and the adventures and stresses that her body has undergone, the scars of trauma, the changes of childbirth, her distinguishing characteristics, the light in her expression.

Bruce concurred, and elaborated:

One of the reasons men like a variety of women is that they would be intimidated if all women were thin models. It's so often the imperfections that men fall in love with. I mean, those models are OK to look at, but they've got no person-ality, lying there on the paper, have they? Your love has got to have something individual to hold on to, otherwise you're going to get bored very quickly.

A man quoted by Shere Hite:

[She] should be quick to smile and enjoy life ... I know several model-like-looking women who have rather dead pans and little expression, which turns me off.

So what is it, if not simply the shape of her body, that gives a woman sex appeal? Many things were cited: not so much individual elements like face, legs, hair colour, etc., as the whole effect, the 'style', 'the sort of woman she is – the aura she creates'. And, coming up very high on the list, confidence.

The confidence to be a woman and not always to be trying to be somebody else.

I agree. Every woman looks her best when she looks proud of herself.

I've often noticed that the most attractive women – you know, those ones that men throw themselves off bridges for – are not always that pretty. But they've got that lusty confidence in themselves and their sexuality that is absolutely riveting. A man just feels dizzy in the face of it.

Sex, Sex, Sex

You think sex'll be better if you've lost a lot of weight?
   Forget it!
   In my previous book, *Women's Pleasure or How to Have an Orgasm as Often as You Want*, I cited the fact that according to the seven thousand-plus men of all ages questioned by the sex researcher Shere Hite, men's greatest complaint about women is that they don't want sex often enough. There is increasing evidence to suggest that larger women desire sex more frequently than thinner women because of the greater quantities of the hormone oestrogen in their bodies. This is backed up by research in America: 'The evidence seems to suggest, and common sense would con-

firm,' writes Roberta Seid in *Never Too Thin*, 'that a hungry, under-nourished animal is less, not more, interested in the pleasures of the flesh.' Naomi Wolf cites a study conducted at Michael Reese Hospital in Chicago in which plump women, on scales of erotic excitability and readiness, outscored thin women by almost two to one.

Several men I spoke to remarked that women who were above the average weight were often better in bed. Tom, after many years of experience, found that

> the reason is that many women who are thin are constantly worrying about staying that way and so always dieting and fussing about this bit and that bit of their bodies. But fatter women are less bothered. They just want to have fun. The thin women I've known who really enjoyed sex usually seem to be naturally thin.

Will Self:

> Big women can haul me upstairs and throw me into bed when I'm too plastered to do it myself – another reason why I adore them!

At the opposite end of the scale, it is well known that extremely thin women lose their sex drive. In popular culture up until the last few decades, plumper women were regarded as being more sexually forthcoming. The country girl who is ready and eager for a romp in the hay is always traditionally the voluptuous one, while her thinner sisters are colder and more remote. Of course this is a completely unscientific way to assess sexuality, but it is quite plausible that centuries of existence without the clutter and intrusion of constant new theories enabled our ancestors to draw accurate conclusions based on nothing more than simple obser-vation. Now – with laboratories to test hormone levels – it seems that they were right. In similar fashion, for centuries a certain amount of flesh was considered beneficial to good health, and a protection against disease. Now, if you turn to Chapter 5 you will read that at last scientists are realizing the truth of this view as well.

If, with a group of men, you bring up the subject of women's bodies in the bedroom, you get an immediate, almost unanimous response along the following lines:

What makes a woman really sexy in the bedroom is, above everything else, her willingness, her apparent enjoyment of sex.

There's no question in my mind that the woman who is passionate in bed, who seems to really enjoy it, is worth a dozen perfect figures.

Of course, talking to women today, many of them point out that feeling that they are too fat in bed is the only inhibiting factor to their wholehearted enjoyment of sex. This might be justification for a diet, if diets worked. It's not easy to get rid of inhibitions about your bottom being too big, or your bosoms the wrong shape, or suddenly to feel self-confidence in a situation (i.e. bed) where previously you had none – but it is more profitable to work on your attitude than to be obsessed with dieting. One of the most forceful opinions I got from men is that it's extremely *un*sexy for women to cower under the bedclothes, try to hide their figure and generally emanate a lack of self-confidence:

A woman who is proud of her body – whatever the shape – is extremely sexy. You know the sort of thing: flinging off her top, challenging you to come and get her, walking around uninhibited.

For self-conscious situations in bed there's no substitute for a good bottle of booze (though don't drink too much if you're likely to have trouble with orgasm: booze is a bit of a killer in this respect). Clothes are very helpful too, and partly clothed sex can be most satisfactory. I personally think a simple man's shirt (the kind that dips at the bottom if possible, rather than cut straight across) is extremely sexy on women of any shape or size, and has the added advantage of buttons that can be undone according to taste.

Every shop in England now seems to stock elaborate fancy underwear (can anyone tell me why on earth those things are called 'teddies'?). Some of it's attractive, but much of it is a lot less sexy than ordinary clothes. As one chap put it to me:

When you see a girl wearing all that paraphernalia it's as if she's saying 'Right, sex please now'. It sort of takes away the spontaneity and makes me feel that I'm being told to perform.

Also, a lot of women find fancy underwear quite uncomfortable – with stockings and suspenders there are all those bits to cut into you – and wear it because they think it will please the man, which is quite the wrong way to go about things. So: make sure whatever you wear in bed pleases *both* of you. That's not a lot to ask, and it's far better than you being made to feel more silly and inhibited than ever, which is often the result of a man buying for his wife little 'frilly do-dahs from a mail order catalogue' (as another man I spoke to described them).

And, to end on a more sobering point, let's hear from Avril:

> In my experience, what men find sexy in the way of clothes are often the very things that women consider most *un*sexy. The other night, getting ready for bed, my boyfriend came in and caught me standing in nothing but my bra and tights. I mean *tights* – how ghastly can you get? But he went wild!

So Why Are Women Always Told that Only Slim is Sexy?

The crucially important word in this subtitle is 'women'. We are perpetually inundated by images of thin, sinewy women – those thin, sinewy women whom men are all supposedly drooling over. But most of these images appear in fashion and beauty magazines and in beauty advertisements such as those for soap, shampoo, face creams, stockings, make-up. You see them on the catwalk, wearing high-fashion clothes, or in your favourite journal modelling high-street collections. Yes, they appear in male-oriented ads for products such as cars and aftershave, but the great majority of these images appear in products aimed for *female* consumption.

The insistence on thinness as essential to beauty and sexual attractiveness is not the result of a careful study of men's desires, but an artificial insistence by advertising and magazines. It is the result of fashion. If you're a fashion victim, then, of course, dieting is what you have to do to keep up. Just don't let it be taken as anything more serious than that, certainly not as far as men are concerned. 'But,' objected Nora, 'if you ask a man – any man – to name his ideal woman, whether she's glamorous or not she's always thin: Jacqueline Bisset, Meryl Streep, and so on.' Of course she is, for the very simple reason that all glamorous role models are thin. There aren't others, because those who call the shots do not allow it. Kathleen Turner was told bluntly, 'You're too fat to be a star.' Being famous and glamorous *entails* being thin, and stories abound of stars whose careers tumble after gaining weight. The men who idolize Michelle Pfeiffer are responding to the beauty and glamour, not the thinness per se. Obviously, the models in the adverts and on the box have nice bodies, but what makes them nice is their proportion and faces, not their thinness. The models in erotic photographs taken at the turn of the century also have gorgeous bodies, and are not in the least bit thin: I have in front of me Serge Nazarieff's book of stereo nudes taken between 1850 and 1930 – not more than one or two are less than a size 16, even including those taken during the Twenties, the first wave of the slimming craze.

Many men I spoke to regarded the women's magazines' obsession with dieting as baffling and absurd:

I can't understand it. Looking at some women's magazines you'd think all women were interested in was sex and diets. That's all it ever is – how to get more fucks by eating less food. Thank heavens, I've yet to meet a woman who's as mindless as some of those mags make them out to be.

Even men who love the stereotypes drew a clear line between admiring a model and expecting their own partner either to be like that model or to *try* to be like her:

I adore Cindy Crawford. She's the best thing since sliced bread. My girlfriend looks nothing like her, and I love her no less for it. If I met Cindy Crawford I'd probably blush and run away.

Susan gawps at Tom Cruise and I believe she loves me. I gawp at Goldie Hawn and I *know* I love Susan. The sad thing is, I've noticed, Susan worries that she doesn't look like Goldie Hawn, whereas it doesn't bother me terribly that I don't look like Tom Cruise. That's the difference between being a man and being a woman nowadays, I suppose. Women take their role models much too seriously.

But What About the Men Who Tell Women to Diet?

I'm not denying that there is a whole category of men who put women down for being other than fashionably shaped. And note, I say fashionably shaped, not thin, because you can bet your last penny that these men's tastes will follow fashion slavishly. Their motives have to be looked at very carefully. I break such characters down into three types:

a) **The Purist**: the man who really does like only one type of figure. He simply won't fancy you unless you're thin, and once you're together he'll start nagging you the moment you put on half a pound. Nothing more to be said about him, really, except that he's extremely rare. Most men who purport to have rigid views on women's shapes are either prepared to be completely contradictory when Miss Right comes along, or are really victims of peer pressure.

b) **The Patsy**: this man is concerned with his image. He wants his women skinny so his mates will know he can make a fashionable catch. He's quite likely to have a silly sort of car (brrom, bbrrroom) for the same reason. In extreme cases he might also have a Rottweiler and a small willy. Such men are essentially weak, but they are also numerous. Once they've nabbed their fashion accessory, they're inclined to say things like 'Of course, looks don't mean anything to me, it's the inner self that's important.' Men in groups are much more likely to succumb to peer pressure than men on their own, so if your man appears like this in public, you might be kind enough to give him the benefit of the doubt in private (I wouldn't).

The trouble is, decent men can be influenced by fashion, even when it's actually contrary to their true desires. The following quotes are all from men:

I'm certainly not claiming all men secretly yearn for huge women. What I'm saying is that the pressures on men to go for very thin women are great. If only large women got just a bit more media exposure – modelling in magazines for example, or advertising glamorous products on TV instead of dishcloths and loo cleaners (come to think of it, they don't even do that . . .) it would liberate a lot of men to admit that they like FLESH on women.

You know, I honestly believe many men don't go for big women simply because it has never occurred to them. You never see anyone larger than a broom handle in a glamorous situation, and so often large women hide themselves away. I know I'm suggestible to what I see all the time . . .

Young men in particular are desperate not to stand out by having an 'odd' girlfriend. It takes a lot of confidence.

When I was young I always went for the girl with the fashionable shape, because I was low in confidence myself. I wasted twenty years going out with women who didn't really please me, until at last I met my beautiful wife and realized what I'd been missing.

c) And now we come to **The Groucher.** Most men who criticize their partner about her figure are really criticizing something else. Such behaviour is an indication that something is slightly askew in the relationship rather than with your body. Dieting and weight are such sensitive points with most women, that they become a good subject for a man to focus on if he's feeling discontented on some other score. Fran told me about one classic incidence of this:

We'd been getting along terribly well when one day Gary started getting cross at me about being so bad at sticking to my diet. He got really nasty and made remarks about my weight. I thought it was a bit strange since my weight's hardly changed and he'd been quite happy about it when we first met. Eventually I found out what the problem was. He thought I'd been flirting with the neighbour and he was jealous and wanted to get his own back.

Vaughan, a fitness instructor, says that he sometimes catches himself being unpleasant to his girlfriend Beth because I get annoyed by the on-again, off-again stuff. If she just said once and for all that she wasn't going to diet, then that would be OK. It's this vow to diet and then furtively breaking it the next day. It's maddening.

Because dieting is regarded as displaying strong will power, it will often be the lack of resolve that's being criticized rather than your weight itself. Andy goes further:

It's such a shame because dieting has taken on such a moral tone that men who encourage women to diet don't do so because they like thin women so much as because they think it is weakness in a woman not to diet. It's got nothing to do with figure and everything to do with behaviour.

So, if you've got a critical partner, sit him down and find out what's *really* going on.

However Fabulous Your Figure, You Can't Please All Men

And why the hell should you want to, anyway?

OK, it's easy to say that when you're thirty-something and feeling either particularly self-possessed or downright cynical. But seriously, it's a point that many worried women would do well to contemplate. At least, I know I could have done with that advice myself in the past. When I was in my twenties, despite being 5 ft 9 ins I never went out without three-inch heels on because otherwise I was convinced I looked short and fat. Swishing into a carpeted room on high heels, my skirts flowing, was delightful. Less delightful was the painful feet, teetering along hard uneven pavements, missing the bus because I could not run for it, and passing through dark alleyways hoping and praying there were no attackers lurking, as I certainly could not have run away.

I did not dress that way only when Mr Right was likely to see me, which would have been understandable. I endured it all the time. For whose benefit? To a large extent I simply wanted to get general male approval. The approval, in fact, of those many men who, had they approached me, or attempted to chat me up, I would have told to get lost! It strikes me now as not only daft but decidedly comic, yet every time I'm in town I see dozens of women enduring the same discomfort that I once did, teetering on high heels, or freezing to death in a provocative miniskirt in the middle of winter, for the same unrewarding reason. And the principle's the same with dieting.

Why bother? Why not recover our dignity by dressing to please ourselves and eating to please ourselves? The desperate attempt to lose another six pounds really isn't worth it. For a start, there will always be men out there who don't fancy you. If you're extremely fat or extremely thin then your shape *may* be influencing prospective partners. But then again, if you are an average size, men who go for very thin or very large women will not go for you. And if a bloke asks you out because he fancies you, then he's not going to fancy you more just because you spent the week in between following Slinky Suzy's Desperate Diet Plan. Obvious, isn't it? And then there's the fact that 99 per cent of the men whose approval you're trying to get you wouldn't touch with a bargepole. So what's the reason for it?

The answer is that many women feel that getting male approval is an essential part of being a woman, that your physical attractiveness is a measure of your worth. It proves you're female. OK, so most of the guys who make eyes or passes aren't worth the time of day, but you'd just like to know that they wouldn't mind finding you in their bed. And the fact that you can't be certain of getting that approval makes you have to keep on trying. Such attitudes are very deep-seated. If I'm looking particularly unattractive and the builder/plumber/electrician/telephone engineer calls, to my disgust I still find myself feeling nervous, as if this nameless man were going to evaluate me and find me wanting.

I've found the best way out of this is to make a clear distinction between looking attractive *sometimes* and striving to look attractive all the time. Most people want to look lovely some of the time, for certain individuals. As long as you feel you *can* achieve it, then it's easier to have periods when you don't have to bother.

It's worth repeating the words of two women I quoted in my previous book, *Women's Pleasure*, because I've had so many letters from women in Britain and around the world who found their simple advice useful. The first, quoted in a book by Sheila Kitzinger, found that while she was pregnant she was no longer regarded as a viable sex object:

Strangely, once I was no longer bombarded with sexual advances, it struck me how in one way it gave me a sense of power, of attractiveness, and, more importantly, a sense that I existed.

The second is Germaine Greer who, in her book *The Change*, tells how on a trip to Sicily she decided, as an expression of mourning for her father, to dress in black with her hair covered.

I found the new freedom from men's attentions exhilarating rather than depressing. There was also tremendous liberation in not having to think what to wear. Black goes with black. One has only to think of texture, of the part of one's clothing that matters to oneself.

Being 'invisible' can be a very enjoyable experience (indeed, I've always rather longed to be able sometimes to wear the Muslim women's long dark head-to-foot covering). After so many years of dressing to please other people it's bliss to please only oneself. And, best of all, when you *do* make an effort it's doubly pleasurable.

As this is a chapter about men I'm going to give the last word to Agatha Christie, describing one of my favourite men of all time – the little Belgian detective with the egg-shaped head and superb moustaches, Hercule Poirot:

Not that where women were concerned Hercule Poirot carried his passion for geometrical precision so far. He was, on the contrary, old-fashioned. He had a continental prejudice for curves – it might be said for voluptuous curves. He liked women to *be* women. He liked them lush, highly coloured, exotic . . .

3

Reveal or Conceal?

She (a model agency boss): There's a growing trend lately
for models with bosoms.

He: Oh, you mean bigger models?

She: No, no, thin girls with bigger bosoms.

He: Are there many of those about?

She: Practically none – dieting always eliminates bosoms
first.

He: How do you find them, then?

She: Oh, all the usual girls are having breast implants.

Overheard at a party

Another major reason why we diet is so that we can look
attractive in fashionable clothes, and fashionable clothes
today are, of course, designed to look good on a skinny figure.
In the olden days a fashionable figure could actually be created
by clothes: corsets, padding, hoops, whalebone, tight lacing, bus-
tles and false bosoms all helped to mould women into the fashionable shape – whatever that happened to be.

These days we read with horror of the things that our ancestors
put up with – stays so tightly laced that their wearers swooned,
and such like. Yet more and more women today, in our liberated
age, are prepared to endure much greater and more intrusive
punishment than that for the sake of looking 'right'. Now it is no
longer merely our clothes but our very bodies that are adjusted:
starved, cut about and subjected to implants and liposuction.
Cindy Jackson ('I've got a genius IQ'), now famous for the extent
to which she was prepared to adjust her body to be fashionable,
spent £30,000 on eighteen surgical operations over a period of

five years. Beginning with an operation to have her eyes widened, she went on to have liposuction on her jaw line, abdomen, knees and thighs, followed by a facelift, two chemical peels, silicone breast implants, two nose operations, a temple lift, lower eye revision, permanent upper-lip enlargement, more liposuction on hips, thighs and knees, plus 'minor' procedures.

More than ever before, women today have a love–hate relationship with clothes. The variety of styles, colours and fabrics is greater than ever, but clothes today cannot provide us with a fashionable figure. Revealing more than they conceal, they are a source of worry for anybody who is influenced by the endless pressure to be the right shape. So, if clothes don't suit us, *we* have to be re-designed to suit the clothes. As Rowena put it:

> Fashion today begins at the top with *haute couture*, and *haute couture* means Claudia Schiffer shapes. Then styles filter down until they hit the high street. The trouble is, most of us don't look anything remotely like Claudia Schiffer *et al*. So begins our frantic slimming campaign or, more pathetically, spending a fortune on plastic surgery.

Clothes were not always associated with 'femininity' and sexuality. Only in the middle of the fourteenth century in France and Burgundy was it realized that rather than being loose and enveloping, clothes could, in the words of the fashion historian James Laver, 'be potent weapons to attract and influence the other sex'. Thus suddenly evolved *décolletage*, tight lacing and striking headdresses. By the fifteenth century, 'fashion' was no longer confined to court circles, and since then every possible combination of absurdity has been seen. The excessively restrictive fashions of Victoria's reign, for example, enhanced the idea that a lady should not have to do anything for herself. Waists are a classic example of the whimsy of fashion – they've been up and down like yoyos. Although a small waist has long been admired, in previous centuries this could be achieved quite cunningly, by the use of horse-hair pads, for example, attached above the buttocks to exaggerate the hips. Enormous sleeves gave a similar effect. Laver has made the interesting connection that a waist in the wrong place – be it very high, as in the years following the French Revolution, or very low in the 1920s following World War I – is a sign of social upheaval and an abandonment of accepted standards of conduct.

Interestingly, for much of fashion history, the hairstyle has been as important as the figure, often more so. In the eighteenth century it took as long as three or four hours to dress a woman's head for a fashionable function, and it might end up piled high with cushions, wire supports, plates of fruit or even a ship in full sail (not to mention mice and cockroaches). The following note appeared in *The Ladies Magazine* in 1776:

> I have seen several ladies, very handsome, so disguised and features quite distorted, by the horrid drag of their hair to a height absolutely half as tall as themselves, and so loaded with game, flowers, fruit, herbs, ribbons, pins, etc. . . . that it has really seemed a pain for them to move or speak for fear the wonderful building be demolished.

The concentration on hair does have its advantages however. One of the best features of the punk look was that it took the emphasis away from figure, and on to hairstyles and colours. Indeed, many punk fashions created an almost exaggeratedly unfashionable body shape.

World War I was a great liberation. For the first time women took jobs vital to the running of the country, and brought back pay packets. After the war ended, the period of social upheaval continued apace. Women were granted the vote; more and more of them sought employment and independence. Fashions, in turn, also became a good deal less restrictive: it is impossible to do a useful job done up like the dog's dinner, corseted and swathed from head to foot in hot, restrictive material. Corsets either disappeared or became less fierce; fashions became looser and simpler, and skirts rose as high as the knee. All kinds of shapes that had previously been completely out of sight were now revealed. Suddenly the real figures of women, in all their variety, were on show. But it was not a complete liberation because for the first time the slimming market became seriously profitable, and there was a dramatic rise in eating disorders.

Today we have even greater choice in what we wear: anyone who remembers the Sixties – the obligatory miniskirts – will appreciate the bliss of having the choice of where to wear your hemline. Yet once again, the incredible skimpiness of some clothes, plus the fact that they all seem designed for supermodels, makes the range of styles deceptive. What woman – even the most slender – has not felt a little anxious at the approach of the summer holiday: will I look OK in my bikini? Am I too fat? Are my proportions right? Have I shaved my bikini line? What about my stretch marks, or my appendix scar? (Among my collection of old snapshots from the inter-war years, many show holiday scenes – the people are all having such a carefree time, jumping around and laughing, in swimsuits that reveal modest amounts of flesh. What a contrast to the rows of humourless human kebabs, solemnly perfecting their boring old suntans, and trying to impress each other, that are typical of beaches today.)

For those of us not prepared to go to the lengths of self-mutilation, there is a whole battery of fashion tricks we can use in our desperation. The drive to look thinner, regardless, has often a profound ring of pathos about it. Shelley Bovey, in her sharp and extremely funny book *Being Fat Is Not a Sin*, cites advice given in a local paper for how 'outsize' women with 'fruity' figures should dress to get 'the silhouette of a long triangle, beginning with wide boxy shoulders and skimming all the bulges to a point at your toes'. To achieve this bodily divorce you're to wear vertical lines (never horizontal, except above the bust), not to tuck in, not to use frills or gathered or belted clothes, always to have limited colours, tending to the dark, and shoulder pads, though don't mix patterns and textures and don't wear bulky fabrics or loose-cut woollies, either. Having made us feel that come hell or high water we must disguise our shape, the article has the gall to conclude that the main thing is to 'feel good about yourself; size is so unimportant'.

> When I had picked myself up from the floor (where I had descended in a crumpled heap with laughter) [writes Bovey]
> I immediately wanted to wear a cotton striped (horizontal, of course) top with masses of pintucks, smocking, gathers and frills, a wide waist belt and a skirt of entirely different colour, pattern and texture, with as much clutter as I could find.

Most people wish to be physically admired, but this systematic hiding away of bodies that have nothing wrong with them, other than that they don't fit in with the prevailing fashion, simply makes one more obsessed than ever. We need to bolster our confidence by wearing what we *like*: colours that cheer us and shapes that are comfortable. I'm not suggesting that a fifteen-stone woman dons a tiny miniskirt, but that constantly 'camouflaging' ourselves is debilitating in exactly the same way that constantly counting calories cancels any pleasure we might take in food. Thinness suits some people, and not others. Ultra-thinness suits very few. We need to shift the emphasis away from dressing only to 'look thinner', and towards dressing to look and feel our best.

Never before have women had so much to offer the world. We cannot let it become a place in which we feel so oppressed by our bodies that even the possible future queen of England, one of the most admired people in the world, suffers from a potentially lethal eating disorder. We must battle to celebrate our strength, variety and uniqueness, and we must make the fashion world celebrate it with us.

So, let's begin not with clothes, but without them . . .

Nudity

How I deplore the substitution of suspenders and silk knickers for garters and drawers. Nothing is left to the imagination. And Italy is far worse. Flappers by the score with nothing on but legless bathing drawers such as only little boys wear in England!

So wrote the poet and philanderer Herbert Horne at the turn of the century. My great-aunt recorded the following delightful conversation that she overheard as a child. It was between a vicar and his teenage son James, who, much against the father's better judgement, has been allowed to visit a new and risqué play.

'I was convinced,' said the vicar, 'that no cursing or swearing could possibly assault the ears, and that nothing was to be seen there that would offend the eye.'
James glanced up, laughing.
'How about the fat fairy? She was fifty if she was a day, and her skirts did not conceal her calves.'
The vicar brought his hand down upon the table with a thud.
'Be silent, sir! We do not mention a lady's legs at table. I presume you referred to her ankles.'

How times have changed. The allure of secrecy, hint and suggestion is gone. Today the message everywhere is that if you want to be sexual and feminine, you should expose as much of yourself as possible. As the first buds open, bunnies romp and birds lay eggs, females of the human species become abruptly extra-critical of their bodies and start madly exercising and cutting calories. Magazines pander to it with monotonous regularity. Week after week it's 'Get into shape for summer', 'Tone up and firm in fifteen minutes', and so forth.

These features only create more anxiety, as Maeve pointed out:

> When I saw 'Three Day Swimsuit Diet' recently, my first thought was *three days* – I'd need three months to look even faintly decent in a swimsuit. That diet somehow conjured up thousands of gorgeous readers who were only centimetres away from perfection.

The perpetual enticements to expose ourselves create a vicious logic – a sexy, fun-loving woman is an exposed woman, but woe betide any non-slim woman who exposes herself. Therefore (runs the implication) unless you're semi-naked and slim you're not much fun and certainly not sexy. OK, most of us feel we can ignore most of these blandishments, but inevitably something sinks in, enough to prevent us being totally relaxed about our bodies. A lot of us would be spared a lot of anxiety if we simply stopped and asked ourselves a simple question: Do I really *want* a suntan? Like thinness, suntans are blindly assumed to be attractive and desirable. I have had one once in my life, and it did not suit me. A lot of people actually look much worse with blotchy bits of brown and red all over them (faces are the hardest part to get right). Skin cancer is increasing dramatically, and the most ageing thing you can do to your skin is tan it regularly.

I adore pale skin and do everything in my power to avoid the sun. On holiday in Kenya recently I attracted bemused glances from the rows of boiled lobsters on the beach as I unashamedly ran into the sea fully clothed in calf-length black leggings and a tee-shirt. Believe me, wet tee-shirts (especially with nothing on underneath) can be every bit as sexy as a bikini – and much less anxiety-inducing on the figure front!

At the same party at which the model agency boss whom I quoted in this chapter's epigraph was holding forth, I noticed that over half of the women present were all dressed alike, in skimpy minidresses. Now, I've got no objection to skimpy minidresses, though I have no desire to wear one myself; but the impression I got was that these women were much more interested in competing with each other over the length/slenderness/brownness/cellulite-freeness of their legs, than in wearing a garment they particularly liked.

I blame the Hollywood Mentality: the frantic need to *prove* that you're in fashionable nick. Jane Seymour's wedding, featured in *Hello!* a year or so back, showed the bride not simply thrusting her legs at the camera ('If you don't show them, dear, people might think they've got fat, or riddled with varicose veins'), but halfway through the ceremony actually removing her skirt altogether. Glamorous models/actresses/film stars who have reached their forties and still look marvellously attractive are forever speaking volubly about their 'serenity' and 'confidence'. That's all very nice, but why do they always pose half-naked, in a wet tee-shirt in the sea, while they're saying it? There's a kind of desperation about it all, for surely true confidence in your forties is better expressed sitting reasonably covered in a chair and *knowing* that you look good, without having to *prove* it.

Clearly a woman who reveals a lot of leg, back, cleavage or midriff will attract a lot of crude sexual attention, and perhaps that is the main aim of film stars and models, but many of the men I spoke to agreed that women who dressed like this lacked a more enduring sexual mystery:

> I'm getting tired of women flashing their legs everywhere. There's a sort of mindlessness about it. It's so much sexier when a woman has style and self-possession enough to keep her body to herself rather than offering it on display at the slightest possible opportunity as if it were a Sainsbury's dish.

> How much sexier is the idea of a calf-length skirt – no legs staring at you, but a graceful swish as she crosses her legs, an enticingly brief flash of cleavage as she leans over. The thrilling thought that you may never know more, unless she falls for you of course. Now there's an incentive to please her!

> I get a kick out of thinking that my girlfriend's beautiful,

47

curvaceous figure is for me alone to see – not thrown at unwilling viewers.

I do wish women would not bare their flesh so. A woman with a very low-cut dress or short skirt is not necessarily sexy but you can't help looking. She's obviously daring you to look. It's so superficial. If a man was walking around with a skirt to just below his crotch, I'd do the same thing. Nothing sexual in it.

At the other end of the scale are big women who strip off and don't give a damn, and these people I support with all my soul because it is not slavish but defiant, and takes a huge amount of courage.

Let's finish this section on a delightful comment from a man, quoted by Shelley Bovey:

My wife has put on a lot of weight – gone from eight to seventeen stone in ten years. She is marvellously attractive, does not want to diet and would not be seen dead in any of these clothes that are meant to be flattering, whatever that means. Wearing a bikini in Italy last summer, she had no shortage of admirers. I find nothing so tedious as a load of women yakking on about their latest diets.

But Dieting Is Easy for the Fashion Models, Isn't It?

No.

R. Swift, Cambridge

All this is very rousing, you might say, but if it's easy enough for fashion models to look good in fashionable clothes by a bit of dieting, then it ought to be easy enough for me, too. I have only myself, not fashion, to blame.

Don't I know that line of thought well! Women feel constantly guilty about their bodies and their lack of will. The truth is, dieting is just as much misery for models as it is for the rest of us. The only difference is that whereas they can get paid hundreds of thousands of pounds for it, we get nothing but a raging hunger. (I'll bet you half a bag of toffees that even the most weak-willed dieter would get slim for that kind of money.) What's more, models these days have to stay so dangerously underweight that they run the real risk of inducing anorexia. The American model Aimee Lui, who herself continued to model as an anorexic, confirms in her autobiography that many models suffer from this appalling condition.

When I was in my twenties and sharing a flat in Chelsea with my best friend, a well-known fashion photographer took the flat above us. He was then working for *Vogue*, *Harpers* and all the fancy magazines, using, of course, the top models of the day. He offered me a job as his assistant, and it was in this way that I saw at close range the life of a fashion model in the Seventies.

The models fell into two types: those who were as stunning close up as in their pictures, and those who you would have passed in the street without noticing – their faces were sufficiently neutral to take on successfully any 'image' required. All were extraordinarily thin, though a lot less so than by today's standards. Breasts were absolutely not allowed ('they ruin the line of the dress, darling'), except for swimwear ads, when special 'curvaceous' models were brought in.

To begin with I assumed these models were all natural fiddle-strings, and I envied them. However, come lunchtime, after a gruelling morning's work (this particular photographer had a passion for making his women leap about for 'action' shots) they'd unpack their rations: 3 oz of cold chicken and a tomato. Without exception, they waged a constant struggle to keep thin. All, before beginning modelling, had been a stone or two heavier than they were now, and had to lose it in order to get work. It was not uncommon for models to have dizzy spells through lack of food; sometimes they fainted. These days they even find themselves at risk of starving to death.

Still, these women I worked with did get paid handsomely (the going rate then was an astronomical seven pounds an hour). Perhaps, given the higher risks today's models face, the now massive sums commanded aren't completely unjustified. It is not only models: I have just finished watching a programme about students at the Central School of Ballet. Each fought continuously to keep skinny. One young girl was regarded with great alarm because over one term she had gained a massive . . . $2^1/_2$ lbs!

For most of us, no matter how much we bant and wobble and throw our legs about in aerobic abandon, we are not going to end up looking like models unless we've already got the right face and proportions. In fact, it's fairly safe to predict the reverse, namely that unless you have the looks and proportion of a model, enforced ultra-skinniness will not improve you.

It's also important to remember that glamour takes time. In the late Jill Tweedie's words:

> It's possibly 50 per cent of what [glamorous women] do –
> in Joan Collins's case, 90 per cent. It's like telling us we
> should all play the piano as well as Mozart . . . to look like
> one of those 'role models' demands a lot of money. And any
> woman who's got another way of spending her life won't
> do it.
>
> *Independent on Sunday*

And while we're on to Joan Collins, let the splendid Claire Rayner speak:

> Women of my age are idiots if they try to look like Joan
> Collins. Anyone who has managed to get her life together
> will laugh at the idea and walk on. If there's one thing I've
> learnt, it's that if you rely on your looks you're in trouble.

Jerry Hall, whose large, strong looks I've always admired, talks frankly about the hours of work, practice, effort she puts into being a model, the oils she rubs in, the constant swimming, yoga, walking, dancing, the twice-daily Jane Fonda workouts, the ninety daily sit-ups – and so on. We need to learn to admire without seeking to copy.

Models who have stopped trying to satisfy the requirements for ultra-thinness speak of their new freedom with enormous relief. Simone Ive of Hammond Hughes modelling agency for plus-size women, recently said:

> When I was trying to be a 'skinny model' I didn't eat a great
> deal. I used to take laxatives. I wasn't anorexic or bulimic,
> but I could have gone that way very easily.
>   Then when I started with the agency they said I'd have
> to *put on* weight.

I'm much more content with the size I am now. I weigh 11½ stone and people tell me it's nice to see a model who looks like a real person, not a stick.

Confidence!

Women who feel they're too large, or unfashionably shaped in some particular, usually dress in dark colours, obeying all manner of fashion rules. Rachel, who works as a fitness instructor, was puzzled by her aerobics class: 'It's funny, but they all wear such drab clothes. Black tracksuits mostly. I can't think why they don't wear something bright and cheerful.' This told me instantly that Rachel had never needed to diet, and patiently I explained to her that women who feel they're overweight have oodles of drab clothes. It's still a standing joke with my best friend, and every time we meet we enumerate all the black clothes in our wardrobes: at my last count it was 12 black tee-shirts, 7 black skirts, 8 black dresses and a mountain range of black stockings.

The alternative to black is loose baggy clothes. I never went in for those, but I know a score of women who have whole truck-loads of near maternity garments stashed away. Rosemary, a 'diet victim and mad as hell about it' who wrote to me from Shropshire, recollected a clothes code she used to use:

> I had a friend called Josie who, like myself, was always trying to lose weight and rapidly putting it back on again. Our conversations centred around this very delicate matter. A not-so-very-subtle secret language grew up between us.
>
> 'What are you wearing?' Josie would enquire down the phone, innocently.
>
> 'Tracksuit,' I responded briskly. I had just come back from holiday.
>
> 'Ah, tracksuit, eh? That's nice. I wore a tracksuit last month. Didn't realize they were still in fashion. Colourful, is it?'
>
> 'No. I'm going through a brown phase. It's much more elegant.'
>
> 'A loose, airy garment, I take it?'
>
> 'I disapprove of figure-hugging articles.'
>
> 'I'm *sure* you do, dear.'

'And you?' I asked.

And to my mortification she would be wearing a blue, patterned frock, which meant she'd lost 7 lbs, according to the code. My brown, baggy tracksuit signified a gain of 1 st 6 lbs; had it been 1 st 7 lbs, it would have been dark brown and baggy; a stone and a half or above was announced by the huffy declaration that, 'quite honestly, I think fashion is greatly overrated these days'.

What matters more than anything if you want clothes to suit you is not figure, but self-esteem. Roger, an ex-fashion photographer, puts it this way:

> What I think is that there is often, how should I say, a misjudgement on the part of women who try to look like the fashion models. They lack 'possessed-ness' as women. Definitely, what makes a woman attractive is her confidence. I don't just mean sexually attractive, but professionally attractive, women you take seriously. Some of the most sophisticated women in the fashion world are not in any conventional sense good-looking, or even slim, but they are self-possessed women. They enjoy their clothes, they . . . stand upright.

Add three stone to a model and keep the confidence and she'll still be lovely. Keep the slimness and take away the confidence and you've a totally different woman. Many of the happy women who wrote to me, and others whom I interviewed, emphasized precisely this point. All their lives they'd gone around worrying about some aspect of their bodies and attempting to hide it or themselves from view, be it weight, features, curves. And then at a particular time they decided to stop hiding, dress properly and put an end to all their self-effacement. Their lives changed almost overnight. 'I never looked back' was a popular phrase.

> As a teenager and during my early twenties my weight depressed me very much. I wore dark clothes to try and slim me down and used every gimmicky diet going. I would not date men because I thought they were joking when they asked me on dates. Frankly, I was miserable. Then, it suddenly dawned on me: do something about my weight or

accept it and enjoy life. As for men, if they were only interested in what a woman looked like, and couldn't see past my weight to my personality, then, quite honestly, the men were not worth it. I started buying bright-coloured clothes, ate what I wanted and stopped trying to squeeze into clothes several sizes too small. I never looked back . . . I enjoy my life, have plenty of confidence, have a good job with plenty of responsibility and have a great many good friends . . . and I am in a steady and fulfilling relationship with a lovely man.

T.B., Lincoln

The essence of those 'before' photos you see in slimming magazines is not so much the size of the woman as the fact that they emanate a lack of self-esteem. Of course, this is quite intentional. A friend of mine who lost a lot of weight at a slimming club and was proposed for use in their advertisement was told to provide a photo of herself 'looking as horrible as possible'. Invariably these 'before' women are cringeing into the sofa, with lank hair, frumpy clothes and stuffing food into their mouths. OK, some fat people feel like this all the time, but an awful lot – including my friend who was asked for the photo – do not. Most of us, thin or fat, have one of these kind of photos somewhere (if we have not torn them up). Imagine supermodel Kate Moss in one of these 'before' photographs: lank, dirty hair, no make-up, scowling at the camera, enveloped in a tee-shirt and gorging on pizza. Not an appealing prospect, is it? Distinctive features usually become ugly when you try to hide them.

Linda, when she's feeling low, applies the Bette Davis test.

Now Bette Davis was rather odd-looking, and not by any stretch of the imagination a traditional beauty. Yet she was one of the most spellbinding women in the world. And what is her distinguishing quality? Great self confidence and firmness of character. Imagine her in a cringeing, blobby 'before' photograph and you have a complete transformation. If ever you're in danger of underestimating the power of self-confidence, try the Bette Davis test.

One of the most encouraging things that has been happening recently in the fashion world is the increase in the number of shops stocking larger-sized clothes and in the number of catalogues – alas, still far too few – which use 16+ models to advertise their clothes. What's more, by virtue of being large, these models often have quite distinctive figures (there's more room for variation) that make you immediately, on seeing them, feel less worried about your own. Unfortunately, many manufacturers who include larger sizes in their range still use models wearing only the size 10 versions, though this is slowly changing. Dawn French's and Helen Teague's shop, 1647, uses only 16+ models to advertise fashionable, bold and exciting clothes. *Yes!* is a newish magazine written especially for sizes 16+, and I recommend that women of *every* size go out and buy a copy. But my favourite publication at the moment is the Ann Summers catalogue. The 'Twice as Sexy' section ('sensual styles for the fuller figure') is an immediate confidence booster to anybody who feels sexiness and 8+ are mutually exclusive.

I believe passionately that if we only had exposure to good-looking, glamorous women who are larger than size 12, attitudes would begin to change very rapidly. We would all feel more confident. I do not mean that all women would want to be size 16 – of course not – but that even the very skinny ones would come to realize that putting on weight need not signal the end of the world. We would all benefit by more exposure of larger women. Even if you're size 8, it would do a great deal to remove the dread thin women have of 'getting fat' and show that gorgeousness comes in all sizes.

With this in mind I have drafted a letter, which you'll find at the end of this book, to be cut out and sent to anywhere – shop, magazine or catalogue – that supplies or features larger-size clothes but uses only size 10 models. Whatever your size *send it now.* If you're bothering to read this book, the issue bothers you.

4

The Scandal of the Height–Weight Charts

The fact is that the tables of 'ideal' or 'desirable' weight are armchair concoctions starting with questionable assumptions and ending with three sets of standards for 'body frames' which were never measured or even properly defined. Unfortunately, those tables have been reprinted by the thousands and are widely accepted as gospel truth.

Ancel Keys, Professor Emeritus at the School of Public Health,
University of Minnesota

In all my many years of dieting it was, of course, primarily my appearance that concerned me. I wanted to look like a sylph, fit into a size 10 and go leaping around forest pools with handsome lovers (that bit in particular) as the women in the ads are always doing. But underlying this modest fancy of mine was the 'scientific' fact that for half of my adult life I was heavier than was good for my health.

At the surgery, the remorseless Dr Bone would tut, tut and peer over his half-spectacles at the dangling, malevolent weight chart that hung on his wall: 'Twelve pounds over, Miss Swift.' (I scowl.) 'No self-control, Miss Swift. You shouldn't be so obsessed with food.' (Can you blame me for being obsessed, I wanted to shout. For the past ten days I've eaten only 800 calories a day, all of it slug food!) A horrid finger would advance towards my stomach. 'Better get that off.'

Doctors and their blasted height–weight charts have such a final, official air about them. By the age of thirty I might have convinced myself that I was truly happy, relaxed, having no problems with nice clothes, men or anything else. But no: that fragile confidence was always shattered by my GP's charts, which told me – in unassailable, scientifically based black and white – that I was 'medically overweight' and that I needed to lose a stone.

This is the real power of the height–weight charts that you see in the doctor's surgery and that are reproduced in every diet book and magazine: they give a massive, incontrovertible, apparently 'scientific' underpinning to an issue that for most women is essentially one of appearance and self-esteem. Of course there are many women who diet purely for health reasons, but I think the majority of us diet primarily because we want to look more like the fashionable norm. Vivienne, a freelance designer, is 5 ft 6 ins and already quite slim, but would like to lose another 6 lbs:

'Health? No, no, it's nothing to do with health. It's pure vanity. I simply want to wear a tighter, shorter skirt!'

'So you never think of health at all in relation to your dieting?' I asked. She replied immediately:

'Of course, I feel dieting is the right thing to do because we all know that thin is healthy. The health issue at the back of it gives an added incentive to my diet. Without that I'd feel losing those extra 6 lbs was a bit of a luxury. As it is the health message gives a virtuous rationale to my desire to be more fashionable.'

'And if it were suddenly revealed that being too thin were actually bad for you?' I asked.

'Well, I wouldn't believe it. But if I knew it really were true ... I'd probably think, oh good, I don't really need to lose that extra weight.'

Sue and Jessica were having a discussion about height–weight charts. Sue, who is very slim, said she didn't think they figured much in her attempts to diet.

'Yes, yes,' responded Jessica, who is a definite curvy, 'that's because you've always been within your ideal weight range. If, like me, you veer between "correct" and "overweight" the charts become incredibly significant.'

I second that. If you're one of those people who's not always within the recommended range, then, try as you might, you can never get it out of your head that even your own body is rebelling against your bulk and threatening abrupt breakdown.

The danger – and it is real danger – lies in the fact that *thinness* has become, in the public mind, completely entangled with *fitness*, and they are not the same thing at all. The following chapters will show that it is far more healthy to be fit and 'overweight', than to be thin and unfit.

Another daft aspect of the height–weight charts is that they vary widely. Not even the scientists are confident about the subject. After my checkups with Dr Bone I would usually wander into the bookshop next to his surgery, intending of course to buy myself a nice comforting murder mystery – something in which the nearest I would come to diet-talk was whether the cyanide was concealed in the camembert or the port. But after a while, I always found myself in the slimming section. I noted miserably that according to *The Food Addict's Diet* I was at least 10 lbs over, and *The Sensible Person's Guide to Weight Control* insisted that it was really more like 18 lbs. I checked a few other books. Curiously, while some offered me a range of acceptable weights, others were intractable, down to the last pound. In some my age was irrelevant, in others, critical (up to 20 lbs in it!), while a third group demanded to know also my frame size, but not my age, or both.

At the corner newsagent *Slimming* magazine ('Beverly Craven Exclusive: My eleven and a half stone nightmare') announced to the world that I was doubtless in the midst of my death throes (13 lbs too heavy). Its rival *Slimmer,* however (perhaps as part of a promotional drive?), assured me that I was okay. But I hadn't reckoned with the Weight Watchers promotional booklet delivered by the postman – *Slimming* was right after all, but that was the *least* I should lose. It wouldn't do me any harm to take off 30 lbs. (Now if that isn't the sort of information to make you dive for the doughnuts!) At the time, I didn't take as much notice of this huge variation as I should have done. The news was gloomy, I wasn't going to start on the slug food till Monday morning (of course); I could look forward to several creamy chocolaty meals between now and then; and that was that.

But when I began researching this book, I decided to double-check. After all, it would be useful to know which of all the myriad contradictory tables was the correct one. So I went to the Cambridge University medical library and searched briefly through a few journals I knew would be helpful. By lunch I was hooked. By dinner time I knew that I was on to something truly remarkable, and as bedtime snack approached and the library was closing I was seriously debating whether or not to hide myself in the loo while the librarian locked up, so that I could spend the rest of the night doing my detective work amongst the book stacks. Hunger drove me out. The next day I started using the CD-ROM computer catalogue, which lists over a million articles printed between 1966 and last month, calling up everything and anything on height–weight charts.

What I discovered amazed me.

Those dreary little height–weight charts that play such a significant role in most women's lives are a farce.

The Case Against the Height–Weight Charts

The history of height–weight charts is long and confused. A study of the folly, ignorance and ambition that gave rise to them would be a fascinating book in itself. I haven't got the space here to do it proper justice, but it *is* important to discuss the issue in some detail. If you worry about what the charts tell you, you should read this chapter carefully and slowly. That first day's research in the medical library did more to boost my confidence about my weight than almost anything else before or since.

In order to keep this confused subject as clear as possible, I have arranged my discussion in the form of a series of questions and answers.

Question: There are many different weight charts giving different advice about what I should weigh. Why is this?
There are, basically, three ways you can concoct a height–weight chart: a) You can just make it up – an unscientific approach, but cheap and simple; b) You can get together a large number of people and find the average weight for each height and pronounce that, for that height, this is the best weight to be; c) You can invent a formula relating weight to height, and say that for every person of a given height, their weight should be related to their height according to this formula.

The difficulty is that each of these ways gives different results.

People use different formulae, make up different answers, or, according to where and how the research is done, obtain different average weights. Hence, there are a great many different tables in use, each with different information.

Question: Which of the charts is right?
None of them. The truth is that no one knows what the right weight for a given height is. There are a variety of reasons for this.

The body is made up of bone, muscle, organs, body fluids and adipose tissue or fat. Over 10 per cent of an average woman's body weight is bone, over a third muscle, another third is fat, and the remainder fluids and organs. However, if you put on weight, it is *not* the same as saying you've put on fat. Muscle weighs about 40 per cent more than fat. It is quite possible to get slimmer and gain weight. I know. This is how it happened to me.

Four years ago a new gymnasium started up just around the corner from where I live. I was already on a strict low-calorie diet and in a burst of enthusiasm I joined and started bashing away on the rowing machines, the bicycles and the static joggers for an hour every evening. For three weeks I lived in a loose-fitting track-suit and never weighed myself – I wanted to postpone for as long as possible that magical moment when I would register a huge weight loss. At the end of the three weeks I stood on the scales and found that after hours of strenuous exercise and careful eating I had gained 2 lbs! A desperate telephone call to my doctor failed to solve the mystery. It was only when, disgusted, I threw the tracksuit away and put on my jeans again that light dawned: they were inches looser than they had been before.

In short, I had lost fat and gained muscle and as a result I was heavier. Had this not happened to me I would not have believed such a thing possible, though among athletes it is common knowledge. But according to the height–weight charts I was further away from my goal. Weight is a rotten measure of fatness. In a recent study conducted in America it was found that weight was only a little better than *pure chance* in estimating body fatness.

Clearly, weight is a rough indicator of fatness in that a very fat person is going to weigh more than someone of the same height who is very thin. But most people still assume that weight is an *accurate* measure of fatness. Not only muscle but bone size and mass are important factors.

Throughout my life people looking at me have invariably

guessed my weight to be significantly less than it was – sometimes nearly two stone less. Whether I was thin at the time, or fat, I've always weighed significantly more than people expect. Okay, friends might be tactful, but the same always happened in medical situations as well – I remember two occasions when I went into hospital for an operation and the anaesthetist came over and mis-guessed at my weight before calculating the dosage of anaesthetic. It even happened when I was a (thin) child. Why do people – even medics – always make this mistake?

I myself often judge people by the size of their face – a round face suggests a chubby body and a thin face a thin body, but that will not explain it because my face is neither thin nor fat. Now I recollect how when I was a miserable sixteen-year-old standing on the scales weeping, my mother used to say, 'But you've got big bones!' My scorn knew no bounds – I wasn't so easily deceived, I *knew* it was because I was *FAT, FAT, FAT,* and my mother obviously needed her eyes tested. Today, looking objectively at photos of me then, I see a perfectly normal-sized teenager, no Twiggy certainly, but no lump either. Why was I always – whether going through a fat or a thin phase – so disproportionately heavy? My mother was perfectly right, it was bone. Broad shoulders and a broad pelvis do weigh more. My 6ft 1in boyfriend and I recently had a leg-measuring contest, and I felt very smug when we discovered that though I am four inches shorter than he is, our legs are exactly equal in length (and no, he's not a funny shape). Now I don't mind in the least being heavy because I have a lot of leg bone. It is not only the amount of bone, but the density that is significant, with denser bones weighing more. All in all, it's taken me three decades to accept that, although I certainly mind what I *look like*, I couldn't give a toot what I *weigh*. And to really clinch the issue, I have just read that the plus-size model Simone Ive, exactly my height (5 ft 9 ins), takes a size 18 dress and weighs $11^1/_2$ st. When I weigh $11^1/_2$ st I take a size 14 dress. The heaviest I've ever been (touch wood) is 13 st and then I took a size 16. Clearly I'm built of metal. On the other hand, Fatima Whitbread, the British javelin champion, weighs quite a bit more than I do, but it's all muscle; I'm fatter than she is. My friend Eleanor, who is roughly my height, weighs 6 lbs less than I do; yet she's fatter than I am. It is possible for an underweight woman with a big, dense skeleton to weigh twice as much as a healthy-weight fragile-boned person.

The effects of this simple confusion are extremely serious. Take, for example, blood pressure. It has frequently been shown that heavy people tend to have increased blood pressure, and so it is often advised that even the mildly plump should go on a diet to prevent this condition. But several recent studies have shown that higher blood pressure is much more closely associated with excess muscle than with the amount of fat a person has. Of course the brawny have a high weight: muscle is heavy. The mistake has occurred because, again and again, people who are heavy – whether due to build, bone mass, musculature or fat – have been lumped together as fat. Further, dieting has also been shown to increase blood pressure. So what happens? A healthy, slightly plump woman goes to her Well Woman clinic. There the nurse advises her to lose weight to avoid high blood pressure, and suggests that she go on a (blood-pressure-*raising*) slimming diet; when the woman comes back to the clinic later – probably, slimming diets being what they are, somewhat fatter than before, and now with high blood pressure into the bargain – the nurse shakes her head and says, 'See, I told you to lose weight.'

There is also evidence that a lot of muscle results in high cholesterol levels. And since high cholesterol and blood pressure are risk factors for diseases of the heart and arteries, it is unsurprising to learn, beneath all the hysteria about fat causing cardiovascular complaints, that increased musculature has also been connected with such diseases. It has, further, been linked to breast cancer.

Your weight also varies according to how much water you have in your body, as is illustrated by a lovely old *New Yorker* cartoon: in the first frame a child is looking up at a fairground sign advertising an 'I-guess-your-weight' wizard (a prize if he fails). The second frame shows the little boy at a drinking fountain, surreptitiously filling up on water to fool the wizard and claim the prize.

In the *Beverly Hills Diet*, Judy Manzel rages against the evils of salt. If you eat a lot of salt, she claims, you put on fat. This is nonsense. Salt controls the amount of water retention in the body. What she thinks is fat loss is in fact dehydration, and the fast initial weight loss on all diets is primarily water loss, not fat loss. Jockeys, who need to be not thin so much as light, sometimes resort to the practice of 'wasting', that is, cutting down drastically on fluids. Their weight drops accordingly but their fatness (such as it is) stays the same.

For women, as you no doubt know only too well, body weight also varies according to the time of month and whether or not you're pregnant or lactating. Remember, also, that body types vary from country to country, even from community to community; that the way the body uses its resources varies from year to year; that the needs of the body vary from profession to profession. All of these factors help determine what is the best weight range and amount of fat for a given individual. Some scientists feel that, if weight charts are to be worth anything at all, numerous other factors should also be taken into account: smoking status, family history, and so forth. Not only this, but they should be more specific in their recommendations: no longer what is the best weight to be, but what is the minimum-risk weight for diabetes, or for cancer, or for heart disease, etc. None of these factors are, or even, practically, could be, incorporated into weight charts, which are at best very broad generalizations; and yet all of them are extremely important if we are to know, accurately, what weight each of us should be.

So, given all these complicating factors, instead of saying which of the charts is right, the most one can say is which one of the charts is the most influential. Perhaps this is the only way to decide which chart we should pay attention to.

Question: OK, so which of the charts is the most influential?
By far the most influential chart was devised for the convenience of American life insurance companies.

In 1959 the Society of Actuaries in America looked at the height and weight measurements on the life insurance policy returns of nearly 4 million men and half a million women, and then, over an average period of six and half years, studied the policy holders to find out what happened to them. During that short stretch about a hundred thousand died, and the data made it possible to establish a correlation between weight and health. The Metropolitan Life Insurance Company then tinkered around with the results a little so that they were easy to understand, and published a chart announcing the 'desirable' weight for a given height.

Once published, the Met. Life charts were unstoppable. They received enormous attention. America, a nation that has always been uncommonly keen on matters of weight, took to them like a duck to water. The year of publication is particularly significant. Ten years earlier and their reception might not have been that dramatic; but in 1959 they gave 'scientific' underpinning to the slimming craze that was just beginning, and that spread like wildfire shortly after.

The charts were revised in 1983, and, together, the two versions have for three decades (so far) been among the main pieces of evidence for the supposed healthiness of thinness and dieting. They have strongly influenced government policy in both America and Europe. That is why it's so important to see whether they're any good or not.

Question: Are the Met. Life charts good?
No.

Among specialists, these charts are *not* highly regarded. To put it bluntly it turns out that the life insurance research was sloppy, the subsequent analysis absurdly zealous, and the resulting figures grossly oversimplified. But the wave of support and enthusiasm for the Met. Life charts was already too strong, and the objections were ignored.

But hang on! you might say. The Society of Actuaries does its research on over 4 million people and then the Met. Life Co. merely publishes the results in an easy-to-understand form – what on earth can be wrong with this? After all, it doesn't really matter whether two insurance bodies did the work or the most august committee of statisticians in the American Medical Association. The data were there, all it required was someone to slog their way through them and come up with the information relating to weight and health.

Question: So, what is wrong with the Met. Life charts?

> As has been pointed out repeatedly, however, the life insurance data are seriously flawed.
>
> Professor Ancell Keys

What isn't wrong with them?

To begin with, nearly 90 per cent of the policy holders under study were male. This has enormous repercussions for the value of the data for women. Men and women use their bodies in different ways and for different reasons. Periods, pregnancy, lactation, the menopause – all of these govern the weight and shape of the female body. And even for the men, as Professor Mann points out in the *American Journal of Public Health*, the information is unrepresentative:

Now who are these insured persons who were set up as

63

our paragons? They were mostly urban, Atlantic seaboard, industrially employed persons of 50 years ago who, in the first place, have bizarrely high mortality rates in the first years after buying insurance. They seemed to know something about their health which the companies did not know. After this rapid dying, the insured died less rapidly than the rest of us – they seemed to be privileged.

Just because the research involves over 4 million people doesn't necessarily make it good research.

Next, there is the problem of how the information was collected. Many of the heights and weights were not double-checked by insurance company agents, even though it is well known that women and heavy men underestimate their weights, whereas light men overestimate theirs, and that men overestimate their heights, while women underestimate theirs. Further, each policy was taken to represent one person. But this means that if a person had several life insurance policies, or let one policy lapse and then applied for another, he would be counted more than once in the data. After publication, the authors of the report were forced to acknowledge that in some cases the estimate of the health risk of being 'overweight' could have been greatly affected by the death of just one person with multiple policies. Anyway, the policy return simply told the insurance company what the weight of the person had been on application for insurance. It said nothing about his weight at the time of death. Even if a very fat person had stayed fat, it might well have been one of the numerous drastic diet plans available that hastened his death. In the days during which the insurance research was done, these diets were poorly understood. As late as 1971, sixty people died from a popular very low-calorie diet because doctors were still in the dark about what constituted a nutritionally balanced intake. Even a mildly plump person might well have been yo-yo dieting, which is now recognized to be seriously detrimental to health.

'But the more bothersome thing about the criterion used,' wrote Dr Knapp in the *Journal of the American Medical Association*, 'is the almost unfathomable (by anyone outside the insurance industry, that is) way that the mortality rates in the Basic Tables were determined.' It turned out that the way the health of each group was calculated also seemed to vary. This was rather like deciding that you'd judge some of the contestants at a fishing competition by the weight of their catch and the rest by the length of it.

On top of all this come the usual complaints about any attempt to pretend that our hugely varied species is in fact a homogenous bunch of clones. The Met. Life charts take no account of musculature, bone density or regional distribution of body fat. And yet evidence now shows that weight on your hips and thighs (i.e. pear shape), has no effect on your health. It is only excess weight around your waist (i.e. apple shape) that is bad for you. This fact alone makes nonsense of the height–weight tables. (More about apples and pears in the next chapter.)

The Met. Life tables also ignore the significant effects of age (even though it has been shown that it is healthy to gain weight as you get older, as tends to happen naturally), diet and exercise. Yet these play a much more important role in determining health and longevity than does weight.

Interestingly, the latest Met. Life tables are divided up according to frame size – small, medium and large – despite the fact that frame size was not recorded on the policy returns analysed, and no one yet knows how to make a reliable measure of it. What happened was that after all the information was in, the insurance analysts (noting, in effect, that the connection between weight, height and health was otherwise too vague to be useful) forced the issue by *arbitrarily* dividing up the results into three! It was decided that 25 per cent of the policies studied came from small-framed people, 50 per cent from medium-framed and the last 25 per cent from large-framed. Simple as that.

And so on, and so forth, etc., etc. There were also complications concerning the period of time each policy holder took part in the study. On average it was about six and a half years, but some were involved for only a year, and others for up to twenty-two years. There were flaws in how the cause of death was analysed for those unfortunates who did die during the study, since for certain illness it is extremely difficult to determine the cause of death. The tables apparently reflect mortality from all causes; does this include those policy holders who died from such things as car accidents and drowning? 'One would be hard pressed,' remarks the weary Professor Knapp, 'to postulate any sort of scientific connection between weight and mortality for such deaths.' On the other hand, smoking was not regarded as an important risk to health and so not included in the evidence. There were – and this is very important, but too involved to go into here – problems about what is known as 'fractioning' the population studied, so that some of the sample 'cells' become too small to be meaningful. There was even difficulty trusting the data that had been measured by agents instead of self-reported, since there are powerful economic motives for a company agent to get an applicant for insurance accepted, and so they would tend to record more favourable measurements than truth demanded. In fact, outside your doctor's office, diet books, and certain, alas, misinformed but zealous governmental committees, these tables 'are seldom relied upon by medical scientists'.

Question: Phew! Is that the lot?
No. There is one last point, which I consider the most devastating criticism of all. In 1987, Drs Ernsberger and Haskew decided to study in more detail the research on which the tables were based. What they discovered is that the tables even manage to misrepresent the poor-quality research on which they are based. Contrary to what the tables suggest, the insurance industry evidence shows that it is healthiest to weigh more than the weights recommended in the tables!

The only case in which the research does indicate some negative relationship between longevity and weight is for men between twenty and forty, a section of the population which accounts for less than 1 per cent of overall deaths in America: severely obese men have a 0.7 per cent higher chance of dying before forty than do lean men. Hardly a mind-boggling difference. The Met. Life tables completely ignore the fact that the research showed no such increased risk of mortality for adult women under forty, reduced risk of mortality for 'overweight' people over forty, and, on balance, that optimal longevity is reserved for those who are mildly plump, and the lowest life expectancy for those who are at the bottom end of the 'ideal' range and below (less likely than even the 'severely obese' to live out their four score years and ten).

Question: But what about other height–weight charts? Surely, there must be others that have been more carefully researched?
Now you're beginning to think like a height–weight chartmaker. Yes, there are, as I said, lots around, and many have been much more carefully researched. But problems still abound. You just cannot get away from the fact that people are not all the same and that there's a whole heap of factors to be taken into consider-

ation with each individual before you can announce – if such an announcement is possible at all – what's the best weight for them to be.

For example, The National Center for Health Statistics, another American body, produced a 1500-page report based on research conducted between 1971 and 1974. I was a teenager in 1971 and I can't for the life of me remember what I weighed. But I can tell you that the recommended weight this report gave for women aged eighteen to twenty-four was based on a total of only twenty-five such women. Twenty-five! There's an example of excessive fractioning for you. The population of America is over a quarter of a billion, and for all tens of millions of women in that vast land who were (or are – the recommendations still carry influence) between eighteen and twenty-four, their 'ideal' weight, the goal doctors are asked to push them towards, is based on a study of only twenty-five women. And these are among the most highly respected tables of all.

Other weight-by-height tables show major variations in terms not just of sex and age, but also of race and income. For these tables it seems that your bodily health depends on what you earn per year, and the more you earn the more weight you have to lose. Get a promotion? Your body knows about it: go on a diet before you contract income-dependent diabetes!

Still other tables, based on the weights of university students, are flawed because – particularly in America – college women are, famously, an eating-disordered population. Such tables might give you a vague idea of what subclinical anorexics and bulimics are likely to weigh, but it's open to doubt whether or not they're much use for healthy young women.

Question: Why do so many doctors and health-care professionals use these charts then?
Given all this evidence against the worth of the height–weight tables as produced by the Metropolitan Life Insurance Co. of New York and their relatives, you'd think they would have been abandoned years ago. The fact that they are still with us reveals a great deal about the youthful state of weight studies, the power of fashion, and the enormous difficulties of medical research of this nature.

The first reason is that they are convenient. Okay, so they are all misleading as they are so grossly oversimplified and some are nigh on useless, but they are still the only means a doctor has of making a snap judgement about a person on the basis of their weight. And providing you are careful, and throw in a handful of qualifiers, they can even be quite helpful. For instance, high weight per se doesn't cause diabetes, but people who are apple-shaped are pretty likely also to be heavy and that does seem to cause diabetes. High blood pressure is another one – it has many possible causes and lack of exercise and bad diet are among them. Both of these can lead to putting on excessive weight, so weight becomes a useful, though *indirect*, clue that there might be high blood pressure.

Another reason is that there simply isn't anything else. It is just not possible to make the sort of mammoth study required to produce charts that would take all the factors relating to health into account. Of course, given the evidence against the charts that do exist, it seems fair enough to say – as increasing numbers of medical scientists are saying – that if that's all there is it's better to do without charts altogether.

Question: The Met. Life Charts were based on working out the average weights of different groups of people. But what about those charts based on a formula? Couldn't you devise a formula that would take all these factors into account and calculate what your weight should be?

Yes and no. There are formulae in existence which are used to calculate what a person should weigh. Dozens of them, as a matter of fact, which is another reason why there are so many different charts giving different recommendations. The most popular of them is called the BMI or Body Mass Index. But you could hardly call it a sophisticated affair. Far from being the brilliant mathematical bit of wizardry that you'd imagine necessary to tell a person what's the best weight for her, the BMI just declares that if you are a 'proper' weight, and divide your weight by your height, twice, you should get a number somewhere between 20 and 25. Or, more tersely, Weight/Height^2 is between 20 and 25 (don't rush off to find your calculator just yet! I'll be coming back to this formula and saying more about it in Chapter 15). In short, no one knows how to come up with a formula that can deal with even one of the complicating factors that make assessments of correct weight so dependent upon the individual concerned.

But why between 20 and 25?

No one really knows that either. It just seems about right for most people, that's all. If most healthy people divide their weight by the square of their height they get a number between 20 and 25. By the 'most people' standard, below 20 and you're too thin, above 25 and you're overweight. Many argue that it should be between 20 and 27; or between 20 and 30; or between 18 and 25, etc., etc. The chart in *Slimming* magazine, if you look down at the bottom of it, says 'these tables represent target weight equivalent to BMI 21–23 for women', or at least it did in June 1993. *Slimmer* magazine, on the other hand, has opted for a BMI between 20 and 25. Bernice Weston, in *The Bank Balance Diet*, puts her goal weights for women at a BMI of 20. Curiously, the organization she set up, Weight Watchers, doesn't use the BMI formula and disagrees with her figures markedly. Even in the medical world these BMI suggestions vary wildly – depending on whose charts you chose to pay attention to, anywhere between 25 and 45 per cent of people are classed as being overweight, nine-tenths of them only mildly so, and between 9 and 17 per cent as underweight.

In fact, the most up to date research from the medical world says that the healthiest weight to be corresponds to a BMI between 26 and 28, which, for my height, corresponds to as much as four stone more than those 'ideal' weights recommended in popular diet books.

Others complain that the formula is all wrong anyway.

So, now that you have seen the great limitations of the height–weight charts you can stop attaching so much importance to them. And remember, it is rare in the 1990s for women to *underestimate* their own weight. Most of us are firmly convinced we are bigger than we are.

5

The Amazing Truth
About Weight,
Dieting and Health

Read the following two quotations carefully and commit to memory! Recite them three times before each meal.

> The latest studies on mortality . . . show that heavy people are as, or more, healthy than thin people.
>
> Wooley and Wooley, *International Journal of Eating Disorders*

> Only extreme degrees of obesity carry health hazards.
>
> Professor Mann, *The American Journal of Public Health*

These both come from major medical journals. They represent merely a sampling of the rapidly increasing evidence that the miserable, droning diet books and slimming magazines have got it all wrong: it is *not unhealthy* to be large, plump, big, tubby, overweight, fat, bear-sized, cuddly. It is healthy to be plump, if you're naturally plump (i.e. if you eat a normal quantity of food and your weight is not due to having spent the last two months in a Dayville's parlour); it is healthy to put on weight in middle age; and it is also healthy to be thin if you're naturally thin (i.e. if your skinniness is not due to having spent the last two months pretending you've forgotten how to eat). But the worst thing you can do for your mental and physical wellbeing is become an unnatural skinny by going on a calorie-pinching diet.

Don't forget that I come from a whole family of healthy skinnies, and was a most sceptical reader. Yet I am convinced.

Still don't believe me? Read on.

Weight and Life Expectancy

In 1948 doctors in America began what has become one of the most frequently cited studies of disease in the medical literature. For over thirty years the doctors investigated the changes in health of 5,127 residents of a city called Framingham, in Massachusetts, by means of repeated, detailed medical examinations. As time passed and more and more information came in, the doctors were able to discover what put people at risk from certain illnesses and premature death. And as far as weight was concerned, they found that, excluding the heaviest 20 per cent and the lightest 20 per cent, there was absolutely no relationship at all between fatness and mortality. Put more dramatically, what this means is that the average-height woman (5 ft 6 ins) can weigh 3 st either side of 11 st and it won't make an iota of difference to her life expectancy.

Not good enough for you?

Perhaps you think 5,127 people isn't really that many. Actually, for a medical study it's pretty huge. Many studies make use of far fewer. Or maybe you feel that 1948 has a sort of archaic ring about it. But remember that's when they *began* the study; it was continued into the eighties and is therefore an excellent representation of half a lifespan.

But let's look at another study altogether.

How about an investigation of 1.8 million people, completed in 1984, in Norway? This is, to date, the world's largest, most useful, population study. The findings from this monumental project once again confirmed that for the average-height woman, weight, except in the case of the unusually thin and the very obese, is irrelevant as far as mortality is concerned. Let me put the information as a table. For an average-height woman (1.7 m or 5 ft 6 ins), the Norwegian Study found the following relationship between weight and chance of living to sixty-five:

weight of woman	chance of living to sixty-five
7 st 12 lbs	73.0%
8 st 10 lbs	82.4%
16 st plus	84.4%
20 st plus	75.7%

In other words, according to the study, women weighing 8 st 10 lbs, the so-called 'ideal' weight for that height, have a slightly

71

lower chance of reaching their sixty-fifth birthday than women who are nearly *twice* that weight! But if you're really eager never to have to draw a pension cheque, then one of the best ways to go about it is to be underweight. Your chances of premature death quickly become double that of a plump woman.

Sorry to be brutal about it, but after spending all my life listening to scare stories about the imminent and miserable demise that faced me whenever I wandered a few ounces above the glorious 'ideal', I feel just a touch triumphant to find that all along the antiweight message was not only overzealous but completely wrong.

So much for mortality. But what about general ill health? I mean, there's not much advantage in living to a ripe old age if you're going to spend the whole time racked by illness, is there? Perhaps skinny people are healthier in general, even if not quite so long-lived.

Wrong again. Weight protects against illness and disease. Keep reading . . .

Dieting Can Seriously Damage Your Health

A few more quotations to be committed to memory and chanted at regular intervals:

> No one has been able to prove that fatness per se cuts life short. If left alone, 99 per cent of human beings will reach a plateau weight, a set point at which their metabolisms will be satisfied and their bodies healthy. It is the dieting, the anxiety, and the perpetual scrimmaging with food that lead to illness.
>
> Hillel Schwartz, *Never Satisfied*

> Recommendations of weight loss are routinely being made despite evidence that they may enhance rather than reduce risk of mortality.
>
> William Stini, *Medical Anthropology*

> The astronomical death rate of crash dieters who regain their lost weight suggests that the hazards associated with

fatness may be mainly related to rapid loss and regain of weight.

Drs Ernsberger and Haskew, *The International Journal of Obesity and Weight Regulation*

Clear enough for you? And you thought the worst that could be said about dieting is that it simply wasn't a particularly good way to lose weight! Of course, the above doesn't mean that anyone who's spent a day without food had better start drawing up their will and putting their effects in order. But it does mean that if you want to lose a stone or two – and, particularly, if you want to lose much more than that – you should do it gradually, in a way that will not upset the smooth functioning of your body, or else you can end up putting your health seriously at risk. Yes, yes, you've heard it all before, and nobody ever takes any notice of that boring little warning on every diet book to 'check with your doctor'. This really is different.

In Part Two I'll explain how you can lose weight simply and effectively. In the meantime let me descend into gloom and misery a bit further and give you some of the details about what dieting can do to your body. Before giving you the good news, I want to make sure I've demolished once and for all your belief in dieting. I know the tenacity of that belief only too well. But believe me, if you want to be comfortable with your body, whether that means losing weight or changing your self-perception, then your pro-dieting sentiment has to be mercilessly crushed.

So, on with the gory details.

One of the main reasons why dieting is claimed to be good for you is because, initially, restricting calories does succeed in reducing the risk factors often associated with high weight. But this benefit is short-lived.

Improvements in risk factors accompanying initial weight loss have been well documented and include reductions in cholesterol, free fatty acid, triglycerides, and blood pressure, as well as improvements in glucose intolerance and insulin secretion. However, it is rarely pointed out that all of these indices quickly rebound and often surpass the previous unhealthy levels during the inevitable weight regain. Thus, the almost certain consequence of treatment (weight regain) results in a greater threat to health.

Garner and Wooley, *Clinical Psychology Review*

But, that said, does dieting without the 'almost certain conse-quence' of weight regain increase your lifespan?

Again, no.

The reduction in risk factors does not translate into a reduction in mortality. In some instances, particularly when the weight loss has been considerable, it seems even to **increase mortality**. In a study of Japanese in Hawaii, it was found that weight reduction in heavy people was associated with almost a two-fold increase in death rate. Similar results have been found elsewhere. In the Framingham study (cited on p. 71), people who lost 10 lbs or more after a heart attack had, again, a mortality rate twice as high as those with stable weights.

In contrast to dieting, it has repeatedly been shown that exercise and a balanced diet are much more important to good health than weight. A recent investigation of 10,224 men found that much the highest mortality occurred in unfit *thin* subjects; the unfit average- and above-average-weight subjects were about the same; but that in all three categories, even moderate exercise had a dramatic, positive effect on longevity (though the underweight still had about twice the mortality rate of everyone else). More specifically, high cholesterol levels, high blood pressure, heart disease, etc. – all the factors typically associated with high weight – were dramatically reduced by a little exercise. Other investi-gations have found that you can lower the risk factors typically associated with high weight by increasing the amount of fish oil you eat, and decreasing the amount of meat, fat, sugar and salt. People who eat a lot of fast food do put on weight, particularly after their twenties, but it is probably because the food is high in salt, sugar, fat and meat that such people are inclined to high blood pressure and cholesterol, and not because the people have put on weight. Conversely, it would appear that the reason dieting often seems to cause, say, blood pressure reduction is simply because most diets are low in salt (a low-salt diet results in rapid initial weight loss by dehydration, so it's a good marketing ploy to keep the salt level down). Salt reduction alone, it has been found, has a much more significant effect on blood pressure than even a very strict diet of 600–800 calories per day.

More dramatically, a study of over 1 million people by the American Cancer Society found also that people who had lost weight in the past five years were *more* likely to die from **heart disease** and **stroke**, whereas natural weight gain had no such effect.

74

In fact, there have been various studies indicating that loss and regain of weight, rather than stable high weight, may be one of the main causes of heart disease. In 1942, the Germans besieged Leningrad and cut off most of the city's food supplies. The number of hospital cases relating to high blood pressure fell from 10 per cent to 2 per cent. But when food became available again two years later, 50 per cent of all hospital cases were related to high blood pressure. There was an epidemic of congestive heart failure – the form of **cardiovascular disease** traditionally most closely connected with obesity – which struck people of all weights. In America, deaths from cardiovascular disease declined by 20 per cent between 1963 and 1974, whereas the average adult weight increased by nearly half a stone. To quote Professor Mann in the *American Journal of Public Health*: 'Indeed, there is more evidence for a proposal to add a weight pack to improve cardiovascular function by increasing circulatory work.'

'The chief benefit of moderate "overweight",' write Drs Ernsberger and Haskew in their 150-page review of the subject, 'seems to be a decrease in **overall cancer deaths** . . . it appears likely that [it] both prevents cancer and prolongs survival of the disease.' It is reasonable to assume that dieting will take away this benefit. Study after study has confirmed the finding, some even suggesting that there is actually an inverse relationship between weight and cancer in general, i.e., that the more overweight you are, the greater your protection from this category of diseases. Several explanations are available for this. Heavy people seem to have higher levels of vitamin A and carotene, both of which protect against cancer. Animal experiments have suggested that fat also both increases the effectiveness of the immune system and protects against the ill-effects of carcinogens by diverting them away from the vital organs and storing them in the fatty tissue. It was found that pesticides accumulate in the kidney, heart and brain of lean mice about twice as much as in obese ones. And just as weight seems to increase the effectiveness of the immune system in combating cancer, so it also works against **infectious diseases** in general. In a study of men in seven different westernized countries, it was found that 'there is a distinct tendency for the deaths from infectious diseases to be concentrated in . . . the lighter and thinner men'.

Lung cancer, one of the most common cancers, is significantly less frequent in 'overweight' men and women. 'Women at the low end of the insurance tables' "desirable weight" range,' report

Ernsberger and Haskew, 'are six times more likely to die of **lung disease** than . . . women who weigh one-half again more than these tables recommend'. **Tuberculosis** and **obstructive lung disease**, in particular, are more common in those with low weight. A study of over 800,000 Navy recruits discovered that large men were far more resistant to tuberculosis, and two other prospective studies revealed that heavy people were up to fifty times less likely to die from the disease. According to one experiment, **lung function** is at its best in women and men who are substantially overweight: for a woman of, say, 5 ft 6 ins, her lungs work at their best when she weighs $14\frac{1}{2}$ st; and for a man of the same height, when he weighs 13 st. The reason for the improved functioning is that the muscle mass of the human diaphragm (the principal muscle of respiration) increases in direct proportion to body weight.

Discussion of lung condition brings me on to the subject of smoking. The pro-skinnies sometimes claim that the evidence against thinness is skewed by the effects of smoking. The reason that the underweight and 'ideal' weight people seem to do so badly, they say, is that smokers tend to weigh less than non-smokers, and so their death and mortality rates are correspondingly skewed. But this complaint can be readily dismissed. In every study in which smoking has been taken into account, the mortality-to-weight pattern has remained the same. Besides, although on average smokers weigh a few pounds less than non-smokers, the heaviest smokers are usually well above average weight. So one might even expect the effect to be skewed the other way. No matter how people may squirm around to get away from it, the truth is that underweight is a killer, and that plumpness (as our ancestors always knew) is healthy. It is with good reason that the old-fashioned word for plumpness, 'embonpoint', means 'in good condition'.

Even among the very fat, **stomach cancer** is two to three times less common than among the lean. In women, some studies have also found that weight protects against **colon cancer** and possibly **rectal cancer** as well. Fewer 'overweight' people contract **meningoma** (a kind of brain tumour), and there is indication that **ovarian cancer** is also less frequent among the heavy. **Breast cancer**, the biggest cancer killer of women, is more likely among the thin if premenopausal and early postmenopausal. It is only in the late-postmenopausal case, probably when high weight has come on late in life due to a high-fat diet, that there seems to be some connection between weight and this form of the disease. In most cases, diseases that had blithely been blamed on weight are in fact to do with poor diet and lack of exercise. The average modern diet, which is high in fat, salt and sugar, and low in fibre, together with the average person's physical inactivity, is to blame for more ill health than almost anything else.

Pro-dieters consistently ignore the evidence that it is being underweight that causes more death and illness than being even wildly heavy. Instead, in their evangelicalism, they extrapolate from the fact that extreme obesity has been associated with a small to medium increase in mortality, to conclude that, therefore, being even a few pounds 'overweight' can mean that at any moment you're liable to drop dead. You find this fallacious argument cropping up again in the case of **infertility**. Did you know that *many height–weight charts recommend 'ideal' weights that will cause dramatic increases in infertility?* Much more research is needed on this topic, but the probable relationship between fertility and weight can be represented graphically:

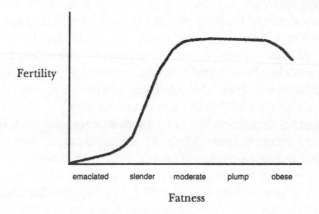

Figure 2
Graph Showing the Probable Relationship Between Fatness and Fertility in Women. (Taken with permission, from J. L. Anderson *et al.*, 'Was the Duchess of Windsor Right?' in *Ethology and Sociobiology, 13*, 1992.)

From the graph you can see that plump women are more fertile than average-weight women. And, remember, the average woman is considered overweight according to many weight charts, even though she is more fertile than women in the 'ideal' weight range.

One experiment found that of twenty-six women with previously unexplained infertility, twenty-four became pregnant after going off their diet and putting on an average of 8 lbs. That's a success rate of over 90 per cent. Just by putting on a bit of weight, these women, some of whom were already within the recommended weight range of the insurance company tables, cured a condition which had defied all other proffered medical explanations. After hours and hours of heartache and thousands of pounds spent on fertility treatments, the problem turned out to be only that these women didn't weigh enough. They weren't anorexics. (Every doctor knows that anorexics suffer infertility.) But they weighed less than the natural weight for their bodies, and their bodies, reacting to this, had no longer been able to sustain a proper menstrual cycle. 'In fact,' write Ernsberger and Haskew, 'the pervasiveness of weight control practices in the United States may be a major cause of recent increases in infertility.' In effect, these chronic dieters could not be trusted by their own bodies to be mothers, because they couldn't even be trusted to feed themselves properly. If I were running a slimming business, I'd start worrying about litigation!

However, you will notice that at the far end of the graph, corresponding to extreme fatness, there is a small dip in fertility. A woman of that weight is still considerably more fertile than a woman who is even a small amount underweight, but that fact is curiously ignored. From that small dip comes the barrage of totally mistaken bigotry that being fat reduces fertility.

Not just fertility, but a less complicated **pregnancy**, with the baby carried to term, is more likely in plump women. Lean women have twice as high a chance of giving birth prematurely, or of their baby being underweight, and up to four times as great a chance that during parturition they'll suffer from **vaginal lacerations**. In a recent article, two anthropologists, Caro and Sellen, revealed that 'maternal fatness [has] positive effects on growth, survival, and reproduction of offspring and grandoffspring'.

Ageing is also slowed in heavier women. 'Pssst . . . it's good for you!' confided a recent *Sainsbury's Magazine* cover, '. . . FAT IS NATURE'S HRT.' Fat acts as a hormone factory, boosting oestrogen levels. 'We slanderously think of fat cells as slothful clots,' eulogized the writer, 'when they are actually among the most chemically resourceful of tissues.' As a result, the **menopause** occurs several years later in women who have not dieted away their natural fat deposits than in lean women. My beautifully thin grandmother once confided to me (in good Victorian euphemisms): 'When I was forty my "friends" simply stopped arriving.' She was clearly puzzled by this early and abrupt menopause, but now it seems that her extreme skinniness may have been the cause. And the higher oestrogen levels associated with increased weight result in less likelihood of hot flushes and the other discomforts of the menopause when it does come. Researchers in New Zealand concluded that, more than anything else, fat serves to keep our bones strong and prevent **osteoporosis**. The chance of you getting a **hip fracture**, for example, one of the most common causes of disability in women and a major cause of death, decreases as you put on weight. In men, the 'overweight' are about five times less likely to have **vertebral fracture** then those close to 'ideal' weight, and the same holds for both sexes in the cases of **femur** and **pelvis fractures**. Naturally, there's no point going through all the body's bones one by one; these particulars reflect the overall maintenance of bone strength among heavier people. Doctors at Addenbrookes Hospital in Cambridge found that middle-aged women on a diet lost a startling amount of bone mass. Only when they came off the diet and regained their weight did the bones recover strength.

It has also been reported that **suicide** and certain forms of **mental illness** are less common among non-skinnies, and (just for the record) **gall stones** are more likely in cases of rapid weight loss.

There are still some diseases associated with extreme high weight. Of course there are. The medical world has not been conspiring with the dieting lobby deliberately to mislead the public. All I'm saying is that the latest evidence shows that the risks of high weight and the benefits of dieting have been greatly exaggerated. Excepting extremes, in the absence of high blood pressure, and providing you are pear-shaped, weight is in no way bad for your health. The puritanical zeal against it was misplaced, pursued, according to Professor Mann, by four groups: 'the insurance industry, the medical moralizers (usually themselves thin), the drug industry, and the docile, unquestioning nutritionists who are too often dupes of the faddists and hucksters.' In this sense, it's a bit like the medical attitude to booze. Not so long ago, drink was supposed to be an outright killer, to be avoided at all costs. Then it was found that, well, maybe doctors had been a little overzealous about the stuff. One or two glasses a week wasn't so bad after all. Now, even as I'm writing this chapter, the latest broadcast is that the stuff's a positive life-saver. I could have told them that years ago!

In conclusion, I quote Drs Flynn and Gibney in *Proceedings of the Nutrition Society*: 'We and other investigators find that in the absence of hypertension [high blood pressure], overweight is not a risk factor at all ... there is no acceptable evidence that relative body weight has any relevance to future health for women in the middle 80 percent of the relative weight distribution.'

There are, however, two more important aspects of the relationship between health and weight that I must look at in greater detail. These are weight distribution and fitness.

The WHR: What It Means and Why It Is Important

The advantageous effects of [high weight] may be greatly underestimated ... since few of the studies cited have divided subjects according to their fat distribution.

Ernsberger and Haskew

The Waist-to-Hip Ratio, or WHR, is the clinical means of distinguishing between people who carry their weight on their hips and those who carry it around their stomach: apples and pears, in other words. Or, depending at what level you think about these things, bums and tums. It's not just a matter of aesthetics. This is a division of serious medical importance, the significance of which has only recently been appreciated. The WHR is shaking up the medical understanding of weight and health like nothing else.

It is gradually being realized that cardiovascular disease, diabetes and certain cancers previously associated with high weight are much more closely connected to how your weight is distributed, regardless of how fat you are. Diabetic and cardiovascular risks are multiplied by six and twenty, respectively, in people with apple shapes. Even if a person is at the 'ideal' weight, an apple-shape fat distribution increases significantly the risk of developing these ailments. A pear shape, on the other hand, is benign. A very heavy woman will probably suffer from joint difficulties, varicose veins and perhaps some skin complaints, but, it now seems, there is no reason why her health shouldn't be otherwise good. It is interesting to note that a woman has about twice the amount of fat of a man. A man with the same amount of fat as a thin woman would be technically obese, and yet women die later and suffer less from the diseases usually associated with fatness. In the resonant words of Professor Vague, the French doctor who first brought the subject of body shape to the attention of the medical world: 'Why such an injustice? The answer: an obese woman is protected when she keeps her [pear-shaped] fat mass, and evidence of her child-bearing nature. When her fat is [apple-shaped] she dies like a man.'

The enormous clinical importance of the distinction between apples and pears does more than anything to explain the radical rethinking of the issue of weight and health that is currently going on in the medical world. And when the truth finally does trickle through it will be the belated understanding of the importance of shape rather than simply weight that will give the scientific underpinning for the shift away from ultra-thin models and obsessive dieting in the next few years.

But how is it that women tend to be pear-shaped and men, apples?

Curiously, human females are unique in having a pear-shaped distribution of fat. In many animals fat distribution is a secondary sexual characteristic, but in none, not even in the apes most closely related to our species, do the females have this particular distribution. There are numerous explanations for this oddity, though as yet no uncontentious one. One suggestion is that roughly 2 million years ago, when our female ancestors stood up for the first time and used only their legs to walk, the previously uniform layer of fat beneath the skin that is characteristic of all primates started to rearrange itself in order to adapt to the new situation. Pregnancy, and the need for a ready energy supply for the foetus, meant that fat tended to accumulate around the pelvic region where it is least uncomfortable. Men, on the other hand, developed broader shoulders, a narrower pelvis, reduced their fat content by about half (the nape of the neck is the only place where fat tissue is normally thicker in men than women) and tended to accumulate it on the upper body where it didn't inhibit movement so much. This differentiation was then enhanced by natural selection.

Another theory – rather far-fetched to my mind – is that big hips and breasts play a deceptive role. Large mammary glands and a wide pelvis indicate good lactation and easy parturition; so, runs the argument, men tend to go for women with big breasts and hips. According to the deception theory, this would mean that women who deposited fat in those regions would also be favoured, even if they had, in fact, a narrow pelvis and small glands, because their lovers would be too dim to tell the difference. Countering this, it has been shown by other scientists that breast volume is not connected to ability to produce milk and that a large pelvis does not mean an easy birth: fat on the hips, buttocks and breasts is what makes for good reproductive ability, and that is why it has been sexually favoured over the millennia. And so the argument about why women are pear-shaped continues to rage.

After the menopause, women are more inclined to accumulate weight around their waist, but, with the exception of those oddities in which otherwise normal men and women have fat distribution of the opposite sex, fat on the hips and buttocks is sex-specific to women: men with surplus fat incline to the apple shape while women, naturally fatter, are pear-shaped from puberty onwards.

Just as it is not known exactly what function the different body shapes of women and men serve, it also isn't properly understood why it is healthy to be pear-shaped, or what causes the body to adopt that shape. But since body shape is sex-specific it is probable that the sex hormones are responsible. The apple shape is largely a male characteristic, and thought to be due to high levels of the male hormone testosterone. The pear shape, much more common in women, is partly due to the activity of the female hormone oestrogen and an enzyme, lipoprotein lipase, which encourages energy storage in the hips. This is why for women the WHR may change during the month. Menstruation involves hormonal fluctuation. Pregnancy, which involves high levels of oestrogen, also leads to more pear-shapedness, as do oral contraceptives, which work by elevating the body's oestrogen and thereby fooling it that you're already pregnant. After the menopause, when oestrogen levels fall off dramatically, women start to gain around their waist the weight they would previously have put on their hips. Hormone replacement therapy, by reintroducing oestrogen, once again makes women tend away from the apple to the pear shape. Repeated pregnancy leads to a high WHR, as does smoking. But more importantly (from the point of view of this book), women with a history of weight fluctuation caused by chronic dieting have also been found to develop an apple shape: 'In other words,' writes Judith Rodin, a professor at Yale University, 'the more often a woman has lost and regained weight, regardless of whether she is normal weight or overweight, the higher her WHR.'

Fitness Is Much More Important than Fatness

The trouble is that the fashion for slenderness has blinkered the amateur and non-specialist medical world. One woman who wrote to me ('I'm a size 22, weigh over 16 st and am proud of it') described the following experience, familiar to many who are fit, healthy and large:

> At my last Well Woman's clinic appointment, 'apart from being overweight', the nurse found me to be in tip-top condition: my blood pressure was 120 over 69, my cholesterol level was 3.1 and my pulse was 79 per minute. There was no trace of sugar in my urine and my lung capacity was 98 per cent even though I am a smoker.
> The nurse said I should lose weight. When I asked her why, she couldn't answer me – after all, she'd just told me I was in 'perfect' condition.

As far as health is concerned, being fit is more important than almost anything else, and certainly more important than weight, which, as we have seen, carries no health risk outside of the extremes of skinniness and obesity. And you certainly don't have to be scrawny to have a good blood pressure, pulse, and to feel the benefits of doing a reasonable amount of daily exercise. The gorgeous Jackie Miller, a fitness instructor of 5 ft 4 ins and weighing 13 st, was quoted (and photographed) in *Woman* magazine recently:

> I'm proof that you don't have to look like Jamie Lee Curtis or Cindy Crawford to help people get in shape . . . You don't have to be superthin to be superfit.

Astrid Longhurst, the fitness writer for *Yes!* magazine is a size 18/

20. Andrea Longden, also recently featured in *Woman* magazine, is 5 ft 4 ins, a size 20, and teaches eight aerobic classes a week. Her ambition is to make an exercise video: 'I've got this image of big, fat me dancing around on TV screens all over the country – and skinny, glamorous women lying exhausted on their carpets as they try to keep up!'

Most of the players on the British football and rugby teams are overweight, according to the charts. So are the professional swimmers, shot-putters, javelin throwers, wrestlers, weightlifters. Is it any wonder that my local gym dismisses weight charts as a pack of nonsense? Sumo wrestlers, to take a rather extreme example, weigh upwards of 20 st, exercise constantly and are extremely fit. Interestingly, a recent study of American school children showed that the most active girls were also the heaviest.

The nuisance is that society is so brutal towards heavy people that they often have little motivation to get (or stay) fit, so that being overweight and being unfit often go together and thus get confused. Leaving aside the brief bursts of well-intentioned activity at the start of a diet, whenever I have felt particularly podgy my instinct is to walk about less, show myself less, *do* less. How many of us refuse an invitation to go swimming, join a fun run or play a jolly game of tennis merely because we feel fat and frumpy? We resolve to diet and *then* play tennis. This is just one powerful reason why we need to put an end to our scorn of anyone even minutely overweight: so that so-called 'overweight' people can have a chance to get fit (and stay fat, if they want).

Amazing Though It May Seem . . .

Amazing though it may seem, many doctors still don't know, and certainly don't appreciate, the information that's contained in this chapter. That's what I mean when I say that we are at the dawn of a new understanding. This material may come from experts in the field who have written papers published in all the major journals, after years and years of medical research involving literary millions upon millions of people; but medicine is subject to fashion just like any other discipline. It has taken time for all this evidence to be taken seriously. The experts know the truth. But the antiquated belief that being even a few pounds above the height–weight table recommended values is bad for you is still constantly reinforced by people not at the forefront of research, including many GPs and even governmental bodies who ought really to know better. To some extent this is excusable. GPs are very busy and their expertise is spread across a huge range of subjects. They cannot keep abreast of all the latest developments, and they cling to the height–weight charts because, in an increasingly complicated and confusing medical world, these offer simplicity and certitude, however mistaken.

Even the fact that government policy in industrial countries still backs up the mistaken view can, again, be fairly simply explained. These bodies continue to base their conclusions primarily on insurance data which, as we have seen, are fundamentally flawed.

In fact, it is precisely because of the frustration so many specialists feel with continued government bad advice on this matter that more and more papers are appearing in the journals noisily reviewing the enormous body of evidence against the use of height–weight charts and the very notion of a 'desirable' weight. If only, they exclaim, people would pay more attention to the scientific studies and less to fashionable prejudice, they would discover that the true picture is very different.

However, all this is not to say that we should each from now on start eating 10,000 calories a day. Some women feel healthiest when they're thin, others when they're large. I know plenty of women who diet like crazy to get themselves down to the weight the charts say they ought to be, and feel rotten. They have not only become obsessed by food, but they've lost energy, colour and enthusiasm. On the other hand, some women swear that if they're a pound above the minimum, their body goes on strike and promises imminent collapse. Neither type is right; both are simply noting what their body is telling them. And in nearly all cases your body is far better at telling you what's your best weight than anybody in the world. If you feel healthy, you probably are. If you don't, then that's the time to start fussing.

Let me end this section with a thought-provoker: in the West we now eat fewer calories than we did at the beginning of the century, but our average weight has increased significantly.

How can this be?

Many argue that it is a result of the bad effects of dieting and others say it is because we are more sedentary now than we used to be. But the most interesting explanation that I've come across appeared in an article published in 1982 by an Australian academic, Dr Bradley. He points out that, since plumpness has been increasingly shown to be healthy, the growing weight of the Western population is 'an advantageous adaptation' to modern food, particularly refined sugars. Thin bodies are far less well adapted to dealing with poisons, and since refined sugars can be regarded as a type of poison, during the last several decades plumpness has been evolutionarily favoured.

Dieting Makes You Thick!

The previously described results indicate substantial impairment of cognitive performance with dieting.

Rogers *et al.*, *Proceedings of the Nutrition Society*

Several recent studies have found that dieters are bad at rapid information processing and have poor simple reaction time and immediate memory. There are various ways these things might be tested. For testing rapid information processing, for example, one method involves getting dieters to watch a continuous stream of single digits on a computer screen and asking them to press a button whenever they detect a sequence of three odd or three even digits. And dieters, it turns out, are pretty bad at it. Research has also found that heart rate is lowest in current dieters with high weight loss, both before and after such tests, suggesting that dieters are less alert and less readily aroused than non-dieters. It is these disturbing results that lead to recent headlines such as 'Dieting Makes You Thick!'

Slimming magazine, as you would expect, dismisses the importance of such findings. In a defence that is truly staggering in its feebleness, under the heading of 'What a load of dieting drivel!', it remarks that 'if this really was the case, then it is likely that being hungry reduced the attention span of the dieters – we all lose our concentration a little bit as lunch time approaches'. So, after hinting that the results might be wrong (or that the magazine has not bothered to check the scientific paper in which the results appeared), it then trivializes them. Even taking the point at face value, we have to remember that slimmers, who are hungry most of the time, do not lose concentration 'a little bit as lunch time approaches' but all day long, often for months on end.

A much more enticing explanation, and one more in keeping

with the sly self-preserving instincts of our organism, is that the brain, which uses up to 40 per cent of the energy provided by your metabolism, makes adjustments when you decide to go on a diet. By interfering with the operation of the central nervous system and reducing alertness, energy is conserved. By devoting more attention to food (the familiar dieter's food obsession), the chances of food being forthcoming would improve. 'These obsessions,' write Drs Herman and Polivy, 'are considered to be the mental equivalent of physiological and perceptual defences trying to make the underweight individual eat if possible.' Once you come off the diet, your cognitive ability returns to normal.

Mental Revolt

One of the most famous nutritional studies of all time was conducted in 1950 by Ancel Keys, a professor at the University of Minnesota. The idea was simple enough. The experiment involved thirty-six average-weight young men who volunteered to take part in an experiment restricting their calorie intake to approximately half of what they were used to. Over six months the men lost approximately a quarter of their former body weight. But it is the devastating psychological effects of this simple experiment, meticulously recorded by Keys and his colleagues, that make this study a classic. Nearly one-fifth of the participants experienced extreme emotional deterioration, some after a weight loss of only 10 lbs. A few even had to be hospitalized. One became so disturbed that he chopped off three of his fingers. After the end of the experiment, the men initially gained approximately 10 per cent more than they'd lost, a number remained depressed and irritable, some got worse, and the unnatural preoccupation with food they had developed during that miserable half year stayed with them for a long time afterwards. This is called a semi-starvation experiment: the men were living on a diet of about 1500 calories per day, compared with their usual intake of around 3500 calories.

The finding of the Keys study that even comparatively mild dieting can, over an extended period of time, cause severe psychological disturbance has been confirmed by later studies. Dr Wooley, in the *International Journal of Eating Disorders*, reports that a 600-calorie-a-day diet resulted in severe behavioural alterations similar to those of people on a starvation diet. Not surprisingly, these psychological effects, however mild, and over which the dieter has no control, contribute to failure. Unlike non-dieters, who eat less when depressed, dieters tend to eat more when depressed. Again, it is the body deciding that anybody so stupid as to start depriving themselves of food needs to be forced back into sense by one means or another. Failure, in turn, leads to further depression. 'Treatment programs,' conclude Herman and Polivy, can 'sabotage healthy self-regard ... All in all, we regard dieting more as a problem than a solution, and recommend extreme caution before embarking on what may well prove to be a counterproductive enterprise.'

The Decline into Obsession

As more than half of the women in this culture today are dieting, this means more than half have acquired at least one component of an eating disorder.
Alayne Yates, *Journal of the American Academy of Child and Adolescent Psychology*

It is now well established that dieting leads to overeating. Dieters manage to stay on course for a few days, maybe even weeks, but then, almost invariably, a lapse occurs, and they have a huge binge. In most cases there's nothing particularly bad about this. It's obviously unnatural and disturbing, but no one would claim that all dieters are therefore budding bulimics. Most women feel that, despite this, they have their eating behaviour under control.

But the fact still remains that, in a significant number of cases, women who begin as dieters go on to develop potentially lethal eating disorders. And, as the Keys study I quoted above showed, the sequence is not confined to women: the effect can be 'experimentally' reproduced among normal men who lose weight.

One recently suggested explanation for how dieters develop anorexia or bulimia postulates that dieting can upset learned hunger controls. The idea is that by denying yourself food, your increased hunger forces you to change your normal eating pattern and increase the size of your meals when you do eat, as well as the speed with which you eat them. After a while, this begins to wear away at your mental control. Some researchers have suggested that dieting makes tasty foods more than usually attractive and progressively destroys those indications of fullness that have been learned during the normal, parentally controlled eating years of childhood. By upsetting these learned elements of hunger regulation, the dieter leaves it up to the relatively insensitive feeling of being stuffed to stop her eating, by which time the meal has turned into a full-scale binge. Other factors may also come into play. If this damage to the learned processes become too great, bulimia sets in, which can result in the erstwhile ordinary dieter now scoffing up to 20,000 calories at a sitting, sometimes causing death by stomach rupture.

And on that note, I end the chapter.

I've had enough of these horrors.

6

Can Dieting *Really* Make You Fat?

How long have you been dieting?
Oh, probably since I was about 20, I suppose – twenty years,
What do you weigh now?
About 10½ stone.
What do you want to weigh?
About 9½ stone.
What did you weigh when you started dieting?
About 9½ stone.

Interview with a habitual dieter quoted by Dr Jane Ogden in
Fat Chance!

It wasn't me Dr Ogden was speaking to, but it might have been; except that I began at 10 st – which I now realize is a gorgeous weight for 5 ft 9 ins. After years of dieting my weight began creeping inexorably upwards. Can dieting really make you fat as well?

Yes.

I remember when, in 1983, the seemingly ridiculous idea was first suggested. 'Huh!' was my reaction. 'A publicity gimmick if ever there was one.' It was also the time the shocking news broke that carbohydrates were good for you. A busy year on the slimming front. Of course, it took a little while for us old-fashioned dieters, raised on the notion of a huge steak and no potatoes, to believe that buying a trolley load of bread and pasta was not a sign that you'd just failed at Weight Watchers again; and, of course, nobody in their right mind would seriously think of giving up dieting. But for compulsive slimmers there were new things to think about. As my friend Josie put it:

90

It gave a new twist to the conversation. It made you lose some of your growing suspicion that diets were all the same after all. Just as at school there was always at least one astrology bore, now at every party there was at least one woman dying to explain to anybody who'd listen the intricacies of oxidation, and the fattening nature of diets. The chances were she'd be slim, short-skirted, glowingly healthy and on a diet.

The year before that I'd gone through a particularly strong-willed phase. I had a friend who ran a restaurant and let me eat there for free – perhaps only because I ate so little. At that time I was determined to get thin – really thin – at any cost, and thus my daily menu was as follows. Breakfast: coffee and a slice of dry toast. Lunch: nothing. Supper: grilled chicken breast and undressed salad. Total calories probably less than 500, and sometimes, just for good measure, I sicked up the chicken.

Sure enough, the weight came off. I felt sick and dizzy a lot of the time, but fired with zeal when my very very narrow jeans did up. Then suddenly the weight loss stopped. Here I was, continuing to eat 500 calories a day, and remaining the same size. Eventually I had to start eating normally, and the weight piled on.

When, the following year, Geoffrey Cannon's *Dieting Makes You Fat* came out, I was on another diet (something to do with mangoes and ginseng, I seem to remember). Not connecting it with my own experiences of earlier, I read the book disbelievingly, gritted my teeth, stopped dieting for a whole three weeks and started jogging.

It was hell.

Stopping dieting was like losing the right to take part in a dear old hobby, not watching the same soap all your friends watched, and joining a peace organization funded by the CIA, all rolled together into one. You just couldn't help feeling that Cannon was a nutcase. All you had to do was look around: my good friend Alice was as skinny as a strip of bamboo and dieting like the blazes – 800 calories a day obviously worked for her. Sarah Griggs, sedentary as a snail and eating about the same amount, looked a perfect twig. Sally Fricker, on the other hand, who ate like a pig, looked like a pig.

Definitely, Cannon was a nutcase. I went back to dieting.

I see now what was wrong. Since that time, Alice has become

anorexic, Sarah Griggs has gone on to liposuction which has left her permanently scarred and suffering from health problems, and Sally Fricker was, in fact, a perfectly good weight all along. She was her natural weight and shape: slightly plump, medium height and curvaceous. She's had more fun than any of the rest of us and kept up much more stable relationships, exactly because she was the only one who wasn't too messed up by diets and self-criticism to enjoy the life around her. And, as her long-term boyfriend remarked recently: 'She looked like a woman instead of like a stretched prepubescent.'

Perhaps Cannon wasn't such an idiot, after all. Since his book, a great deal of research has been done. The problem now is not so much whether dieting does or does not make you fat – most dieters know in their heart of hearts that it does – but *how.* And the answers can be divided into two broad categories that, despite the confidence of Cannon's title, are still not properly understood.

First, there is a physiological way in which the body resists diets and attempts to counteract them by lowering metabolism and preferentially putting on fat during the virtually inevitable weight rebound after the diet.

Before I go on, however, let me clarify what I mean by 'metabolism'. It refers (in the slimming world, at least) to the minimum energy needed to keep the resting, awake body alive. In the medical world it is more precisely called the 'basal metabolism' and it has nothing to do with the amount of energy you use up during exercise or to digest food, the two other main methods of expending calories. It is the basal metabolism which is reduced by the effects of dieting. In the average woman it accounts for about 60 per cent of total energy requirements, or about one calorie per minute, which amounts to roughly 1400 calories per day or over half a million calories per year. These figures are very crude, however: the basal metabolic rate can vary considerably from person to person.

The second way in which the body appears to resist diets is psychological. This includes the common observation that as soon as you try to give something up, you start thinking about it more than ever and the recent, fascinating research that suggests diets result in chemical changes in the brain that may increase one's urge and need for food.

Dieting Makes You Fat – the Physiological Reason

We humans are a relatively new species. About 1.6 million years old is the current estimate. For 1595 million of those years, i.e. for 99.7 per cent of the history of our species, we were hunter-gatherers living always on the brink of starvation. It is only in the last 5000 years that we've become civilized. In evolutionary terms, 5000 years is the merest blip, a fraction of a second. Physically, we are still born to survive as hunter-gatherers, which is no bad thing, since in many parts of the world the food supply is still extremely uncertain, with frequent famines.

It is this survival mechanism that is responsible for our body's response to dieting. The body views any suggestion of extended food shortage with considerable alarm: not as a jolly convenient way to lose a few extra pounds in order to fit into the summer bikini, but as a suspicious food shortage with the possibility that there's an out-and-out famine hot-footing towards you.

Its reaction is almost immediate.

Four hours without food and the metabolic rate starts to decrease. Within twenty-four hours, the metabolic rate may have gone down by up to 5 per cent. If it is a mild – say, 1200-calorie – diet, the decrease will remain at about this level. A more severe diet of 750 calories will result in a dramatically greater decrease of 15 per cent while a starvation diet may cut your metabolic rate by over a quarter. These are average decreases: in some people the effect is less, in others more.

So, you don't have to go on a very low-calorie diet to provoke this response. The body can't take the risk of dismissing your average, mild slimming diet as just a bit of fashionable flesh reduction. After all, a famine can just as easily begin mildly as severely. This effect, the exact nature of which is vigorously debated in the scientific literature, is known as the set-point mechanism, because your body, by adjusting the efficiency with which it burns up food for energy, attempts to keep weight at a set point.

Everything you ever tried, I tried. I went through exercises, rolled on the floor, cut down my food, gave up sweets, fats and starches, wore elastic clothing, tried electricity, massage,

93

osteopathy, vibration, hot and vapor baths, swallowed pellets, capsules and teas – gained as rapidly as I lost.

Lucile Kimball, American inventor of Kimball's reducing powder, in 1914

Of course, by cutting back on the calories you do still lose weight. Your body has to have a certain amount of energy to keep itself going, and if this energy isn't provided at the supper table, then it has to come from the reserves, namely fat and muscle. On a well-balanced, gradual reduction diet, you lose about a quarter of your weight in muscle and three-quarters in fat. On a crash diet you lose over half your weight in muscle tissue. Because muscle is much heavier than fat, this is part of the reason why crash diets result in so much weight loss.

The 'dieting makes you fat' thesis suggests that repeated attempts at weight loss result in a permanent decrease in your metabolic rate. In other words, the body gets so fed up with this on-again off-again business that it decides it's easier to assume you're always in a state of famine risk, and keep your metabolism low even when you start eating normally again. This would explain why, after a diet, the weight you've lost comes right back again unless you continue to eat less than a normal person would. Recently, however, this part of the theory has been disputed. Many scientists believe in it, but some researchers have found in their experiments that the metabolic rate does gradually return to the usual level after a diet. The answer probably lies somewhere between these two camps of opinion; that a permanent reduction in metabolic rate can occur, particularly in the case of people who have dieted repeatedly or severely. Nevertheless, the fact remains that people who stop their diets tend to regain the weight they've lost and often a bit more. It's happened to me countless times. But, one might ask, in those cases in which your metabolism isn't permanently affected, and you eat roughly the same as before, how can this be so?

The new answer is, in part, that as soon as you stop dieting your body starts depositing energy preferentially as fat. It doesn't matter if what you lost during the diet was 25 per cent or 50 per cent muscle, or, it seems, if you eat only a minimal amount of fat after you've come off the diet; what comes back is proportionately higher in fat. The reason for this is still unclear to scientists. One proposal is that it may be easier to rebuild fat than muscle, and since the prime object of the alerted body is to secure energy stores as quickly as possible, it naturally opts for the easiest method. Another suggestion is that after a lean period the body secretes extra insulin to help in the conversion of food to fat. It has been shown that in the case of even very fat rats, during very severe diets they become thinner, as expected, but that they preserve high body fat at the expense of muscle mass and vital organs such as brain, heart, kidney and liver. In the wild, this turns out to be beneficial. In a seminal paper published in the *American Journal of Human Genetics* in 1961, the author termed this ability the 'thrifty trait'. Animals capable of decreasing their metabolism when food supplies are low, and preferentially increasing fat stores when the food becomes common again, are less likely to die as a result of the food variation. And if what you regain after a diet tends to be more fatty than that you lost, and fat is less dense than muscle, then, in order to return to your previous weight, you must have *increased* your overall bulk. Not only do you weigh what you did before, but you're also larger.

Part of the difficulty in discussing the effects of dieting is differentiating between those effects caused by only losing weight, and those caused by losing weight and then regaining it several times over, which is called 'yo-yo' dieting. Since virtually all diets fail and the weight lost is quickly regained, and since nearly every woman who has dieted once unsuccessfully tries again later, it would be more accurate to take 'dieting' to *mean* yo-yo dieting, and to refer to a calorie-restriction programme that results in maintained weight loss after one go by some other term. It is this yo-yo dieting that is particularly culpable in making you fat. As Dr Brownell points out in *Krause's Food, Nutrition and Diet Therapy*, one of the major American medical textbooks on the subject:

We have become a nation of 'yo-yo' dieters – our weight perennially cycling down, up, down, and up again. Still, despite their frustration, few dieters question the wisdom of dieting. After all, they reason, the worst that can happen is to regain the weight they've lost – in which case they can just go on a diet again.

But new research shows there is a risk; yo-yo dieting can seriously distort the body's weight-regulation system. It seems that the more diets you go on, the harder it becomes to lose weight. Even worse, there is new evidence that repeated yo-

yo dieting may increase your risk of heart disease.

During weight regain, not only does there seem to be a preferential tendency to store fat, but also to shift the fat away from its original place and store it around the abdomen. Again, you'd expect this to be because it is easier to deposit and remove fat from this area than it is from, say, your hips and thighs. But, as you'll remember from Chapter 5, whereas fat on your hips and thighs is benign, that around your stomach can be very risky.

It doesn't matter whether you're skinny or large when you begin dieting. It doesn't even matter whether you're human or not. Rats, poor creatures, have been subject to all sorts of caloric humiliations over the years in order to substantiate the theory. It's always the same – go on a diet, and the first thing your body does is lower the amount of food it burns up in order to fuel day-to-day living; go off the diet, and the next thing your body does is start concentrating on the fat reserves in case you get it into your mind to do such a damn fool thing again.

At the University of Pennsylvania School of Medicine, Professor Brownell made some rats undergo yo-yo dieting:

> The results were striking. The first time the yo-yo-ing rats lost weight, it took 21 days for them to go from obese to normal weight. On their second diet, it took 46 days for the same loss, even though the rats ate exactly as many calories as they had the first time!
>
> And with each yo-yo, it became easier for the rats to regain. After the first diet, they took 45 days to become obese again; after the second diet, they took only 14 days. In other words, on the second yo-yo cycle, *it took twice as long to lose weight, and only one-third as long to regain it.*
>
> (Brownell's italics)

Note that the dramatic effects were noticeable as early as the second diet. In other words, only *one* failed attempt at significant weight loss and the metabolism is forewarned. Brownell then decided to study human yo-yo dieters. Looking at 140 people who'd gone on very-low-calorie diets (in which, unsurprisingly, the effect is most pronounced) at a diet clinic, lost weight, regained it and come back for another go, he found that while these dieters had lost an average of 2.3 lbs per week the first time round, they'd lost only 1.3 lbs per week the second time.

Sally, an economist, put it like this:

> You have to think of your body as a rather suspicious, penny-pinching, bourgois housewife living just after the war. She reads in the paper that there's a shortage of baked beans threatened, so immediately she starts cutting back on the amount she serves out at each meal. When the shortage is over, she hurries to the cash and carry to spend all the housekeeping money on a job lot, just in case it happens again and the prices shoot through the roof like last time. As the years go by, she gets better and better at economizing with the restricted product when the shortage comes, and hoarding it when the shortage ends, thus ensuring that, unlike her more profligate neighbours, the shortages come to have less and less immediate influence on the amount of food eaten in her house even if most of the meal does happen to be baked beans, baked beans, and precious little else beside baked beans. She's a mean-minded little sod, the body, but bloody good at looking after herself.

As you'd expect, the idea that dieting makes you fat is none too popular with the dieting magazines. In an article in *Slimming* the idea that dieting makes you fat is denounced. It's worth looking in more detail at the refutation. It's a rather shrewd piece of sneering. What it does is to acknowledge the truth of the claim but insist it applies only to yo-yo dieters, who are those who 'lose a lot of excess weight, then put it all back on again' by going on 'crash or faddy diets for quick weight loss'. You know, the sort of person 'who has lost 8 lbs in a week'. On the other hand, it claims dieters 'following a diet of no less than 1000 calories a day, such as those featured in *Slimming*, will lead to a gradual, safe weight loss, where the weight you lose is fat and not muscle'.

Even these few extracts involve one error of definition and one error of fact. Not bad, for a section that comes under the heading of 'Nutritional Know-How'. First, 'yo-yo dieting' means simply losing and gaining weight repeatedly on diets – it doesn't have to be anything like as much as 8 lbs a week. Even clinically controlled very-low-calorie diets, in which the fattening effect is most marked, can result in as little an average weight loss of 1–2 lbs a week. Besides, how quickly you lose the weight is much less important than that you lose a significant amount – 5–10 lbs – and then put it on again. This may be sufficient to make you fatter, and as we have seen it certainly does your health no favours.

> Dieters more often than not end up yo-yoing; weight fluctu-
> ates as periods of successful abstinence are cancelled out by
> bouts of capitulation to forbidden food. Indeed, there is
> mounting evidence that the periods of indulgence may more
> than compensate for the periods of abstinence . . . Dieting,
> in fact, may be more of an insult to nature. Certainly nature
> takes its revenge physiologically and psychologically on most
> dieters.
>
> Drs Herman and Polivy, *New Scientist*

And as for the contention that 1000 calories a day does not cause
muscle loss: this is nonsense. All weight loss involves muscle loss
to some degree, and 1000 calories per day is only 200 calories
above some medical definitions of a very-low-calorie diet. In a
review of twenty-two different studies, Dr Prentice of the MRC
Dunn Clinical Nutrition Centre in Cambridge, concluded:

> This analysis strongly suggests a threshold, at or about
> [1200 calories per day] below which the perceived advan-
> tages of rapid weight loss may, in the longer term, be offset
> by a more pronounced physiological defence against weight
> loss.

In fact, the only good thing about this *Slimming* article is that it
shows the medical evidence is finally starting to make the dieting
industry jumpy.

Just as the body resists weight loss by making metabolic adjustments, it also resists gain. In a classic experiment done during the
Sixties, researchers subjected a group of very game prisoners to a
diet containing about twice their usual amount of calories for
a period of roughly six months. Most of the men readily put on a
few pounds at first, but then their metabolism increased markedly
to compensate for the sudden excess. One prisoner stopped gaining weight even though he was eating close to 10,000 calories per
day!

The Psychological Response to Denial

Dieting causes overeating. Overeating causes weight gain. Weight gain causes dieting. In fact, dieting no longer seems to refer to eating less. What most people are doing when they 'diet' is a combination of eating less and eating more. They swing from times of restricting food to times of compensating for this restriction.

Dr Ogden, *Fat Chance!*

It is not possible never to wander off the diet.

Dr Leader, *Proceedings of the Nutrition Society*

In the introduction to this book I described my grandmother, Gladys, who lived on virtually nothing. The other day I came across a letter from her written during World War I when food was rationed. Even under those severe conditions, Gladys had as much food in the house as she ever had, but it was the only time she showed the slightest sign of greed. Caught in London with her two small boys, she wrote the following letter to her parents, Alice and Herbert, who were comfortably ensconced in Gibraltar:

Dearest Mama and Papa,

Your offer to send a ham or bacon is too wonderful, we have not tasted such a thing for years. If you could smuggle it by an admiral you would have to do it up so as not to look like ham – could you disguise its shape?

I have a little butter which I keep hidden in a large vegetable dish and bring out when no one is looking. I ate an orange for lunch today and it was really quite filling. The butcher tonight under cover of dark brought a *quarter* of a leg of mutton. He never dares bring it in the day for fear of having his shop raided.

The cake has arrived, it is a simply gorgeous cake and weighs *tons*. We gave poor next-door neighbour some in the beginning and he has been asking pathetically after it ever since.

Luckily the shopkeepers seem inclined to cheat the government wherever possible. I never wish to see a potato or lentil again. I'm sorry this letter is so obsessive, but everyone is getting quite imbecile with this food rationing . . .

Everyone is familiar with the fact that as soon as you try to deprive yourself of something you enjoy you think about it all the time, be it food, smoking, drugs, or extra-marital affairs. Whenever I've been on a diet I've thought about food constantly. I can never forget my hunger; and when I'm full I can never forget that I'll soon be empty again or, indeed, that I will not be able to eat freely even when the next meal is due. Food is calling out to me from everywhere. Whatever I'm doing, I think to myself that this would be a lot nicer if I had a plate of spaghetti beside me. It is not the nourishment I want, but the comfort and relaxation that the forbidden stuff offers. The very fact that I am resisting something that I previously enjoyed makes me feel frustrated. This is *not* because I am weak-willed – as slimming magazines would have you believe – but because I am an average normal, healthy human being. Sarah says that whenever she goes on a diet she immediately thinks of one of her old boyfriends:

> Bob was very nice, very sweet, but he wasn't highly sexed. And just because I knew I couldn't have it, I suddenly started wanting it all the time. I would get into bed with him and think; 'I don't want sex now, but if I did, I wouldn't be able to have it', and from then on I'd be unable to think about anything else. It's just the same with dieting. The only occasions when I seriously overeat are when I'm on a diet, although it always takes me a long time after a diet to get my eating habits sensible again.

Yet you'd think that a person who was really dead set on losing weight would be able to overcome this. Apply an iron will, and she'll get through.

Don't bank on it.

There's a little test that psychologists do called 'preloading'. Roughly speaking, the psychologist coaxes some poor self-confessed dieter off the street with a spurious excuse about doing an experiment in taste perception, shoves her in the lab, and then gives her a 'preload', or, in other words, a tasty, high-calorie snack such as a Twix bar or a milkshake. After the titillating little treat, everybody withdraws, leaving the dieter behind with bowls of ice cream, chocolate cake or similar high-calorie foods in easy reach. Then, pens poised and peering through the one-way mirror, they wait to see what happens. Usually what happens is this: the dieter goes dotty. She abandons there and then the diet she had been faithfully following, starts scoffing, and ends up leaving the lab feeling a miserable failure. This is particularly the case for chronic dieters, whose habit has gradually eroded their self-esteem. Even though it was only a small snack, given to her as part of a clinical exercise rather than stolen in a moment of furtiveness, the result is that she feels depressed about the lapse, angry that she should be made to feel depressed, repelled by the very idea that she should have to lose weight, suddenly more hungry than ever, and decides that she might as well go the whole hog and have an all-out binge. This sort of experiment is becoming a favourite pastime of nutritional researchers.

Women who are not on a diet do not behave in this way. There are various interesting subtleties to this experiment. If the preload is low-calorie, the dieter tends not to eat the ice cream afterwards. But if the preload is labelled high-calorie even when it is in truth low-calorie – say, a thick, hearty-looking milkshake which is really just fat-free milk and some thickening agent – it's odds on that the dieter will break her diet just as if she'd eaten a chocolate bar. In the words of Dr Ogden, 'the foods which dieting has made forbidden cause you to eat more than if you had not been dieting at all. They trigger a reaction. And this reaction is overeating.'

Part of the trouble is that dieting, in the mind of the dieter, is either all or nothing. She can go along for a few days, perhaps even a few weeks, religiously keeping down the calories; but if she once gives in to temptation – a couple of biscuits perhaps – she thinks the whole war is lost, throws caution to the winds and scoffs the whole packet. The common opinion is that it's all a matter of willpower; but willpower is a very vague term overloaded with moralizing messages. Given that dieting is really just a form of self-starvation which your body resists from the start, it seems more accurate in this case to define willpower not as something admirable, but as a bloody-minded resistance to your mental and physiological drive for self-preservation.

Outside the lab, of course, 'preloads' litter the world. As soon as you go on a diet, it seems as if all the things you shouldn't eat have suddenly multiplied enormously in number. We begin well, but soon the strength of our body's natural urge for unrestricted food overwhelms our resistance. Most dieters, like myself, quickly turn into chronic dieters. It becomes a way of life, on again, off again, until, after many years, we finally have the sense to give the game up. It is particularly so in the case of a woman with a family, because hubby and kiddies usually aren't quite so keen on the dieting as she is. Ann Leader, in a recent article, rare amongst academic pieces for being humorous, describes that all too familiar dieting cycle so well that I'll quote her verbatim:

PHASE ONE

'Hope springs eternal in the human breast'

In this phase the dieter starts afresh. The old slate of failure is wiped clean and the new miracle method is taken on board with vigour and optimism.

The person usually chooses some day symbolic of a new beginning, New Year's Day, the first day of Lent, Mondays, or in the case of many disillusioned dieters, every single morning. People rarely start their diets on rainy Sunday afternoons. It smacks of failure before it even begins.

The diet chosen is often new, adventurous and difficult, demanding total concentration and dedication. Alternatively, it may be the 'old reliable' which has proved over the years to produce the most rapid weight loss in the least possible time.

The diet is strictly adhered to and becomes the main focus of attention. Calorie counting is obsessive and meal times are set aside with rigidity and reverence.

The dieter meets with great success for the first 5 days. This is particularly true of the low-carbohydrate diets where water is lost more quickly. The rapid weight loss is accompanied by feelings of power and euphoria.

Often, the dieter, spurred on by success, eats even less than permitted. She believes that this demonstrates even greater willpower and self control. This wonderful state of affairs lasts on average between 5 and 10 days.

At the end of the first week hunger and boredom are setting in. It becomes difficult to get the expensive and exotic ingredient. The 5-mile walk that was light and joyful on Monday has become a tedious bore by Sunday.

As self-pity and misery increase, the old familiar cravings become harder to ignore. The dieter knowingly waits for, even welcomes, any excuse to pull the trigger that will blow this latest and greatest diet to bits.

The die is cast and before reason prevails, the first bar of chocolate is already winding its way down the gullet. Once the gravity of the situation is fully grasped it is already too late and the battle of the bulge is once again postponed.

PHASE TWO

'Eat, drink and be merry, for tomorrow we diet'

The moment the dieter feels she has 'broken out' she enters phase two. Although the initial damage in terms of energy may not be very great, it is the psychological reaction to the break-out that determines subsequent events.

Her thoughts run on the following lines: 'I am a hopeless case. I have no willpower whatsoever. I give in at the slightest provocation. Now that I have blown it I may as well go the whole hog and eat away to my heart's content.

'Tomorrow I will try again and give up for ever cakes, sweets and biscuits. This is my last chance to savour them without restriction.' Now that permission has been granted she can eat all she wants with relish and enjoyment.

By the time tomorrow comes she is so disgusted with herself that she has no heart or stomach for starvation. She stands on the scales only to discover that what she lost in a week of hell has been almost completely regained after a few hours of feasting.

If dieting is this difficult, she concludes, she would rather be fat and happy. She is now poised to enter the next phase.

PHASE THREE

'I am now stepped in so far that should I wade no more returning were as tedious as go o'er'

This is the phase where the dieter makes no attempt to diet. She is angry and disillusioned with the whole business. Whereas before she would automatically zone in on any discussion of food or calories, she now assiduously avoids them.

She stops weighing, takes no exercise, give up the gym and sleeps in on Sundays. She eats what she likes, when she likes. In severe cases she stops going out as she cannot bear to be seen 'fat and ugly' and so obviously out of control.

Food becomes her only comfort and she turns to it like an old friend. She is full of shame and often eats in secret.

Sooner or later she is confronted by well-meaning family and friends. This usually results in a row and gives her an excuse to eat even more. Her weight breaks all past records and soars to new heights.

In desperation she sees the light and is ready for redemption once more. She rounds up all the old heavy-weights and together they sniff around for new solutions. The grapevine is extremely active and is always eager to yield up new and painless remedies.

Eureka! Luck at last! She finds the new drug, the diet of diets, the foolproof method. She enters phase one again and history repeats itself over and over and over again.

Sound familiar? Is it any wonder that we are 'a nation of yo-yo dieters'?

The Neurochemical Effects of Dieting

But there is still another way in which dieting can make you fat; and, again, it is one that has much more to do with the body's overwhelming urge for self-preservation than with the meagre old business of willpower.

Dieters, unlike non-dieters, binge especially when depressed. Much of the gimmickry of diet books exists not merely to make you part with your money, but also to attempt to lessen the downright miserableness of having to cut back on your food. There is, however, a growing body of evidence that even mild dieting has a depressing effect on chemical mood regulators in the brain which bingeing counteracts.

Serotonin is a brain chemical associated with the control of appetite and depression. Crudely speaking, low levels of serotonin are associated with bad mood and increased appetite. The level of serotonin appears to be influenced by the amount of carbohydrates, in particular sugars, that we eat. This is why dieters are noted for their sweet tooth. Unlike non-dieters, they continue to desire sweet food even after a rich meal, a neurochemical effect which is evidence, write Herman and Polivy, of the body 'trying to seduce its owner into excessive indulgence – of sweet calorifically dense foods – so that the lost weight may be restored'.

Not just dieters, but people suffering from everything from alcohol withdrawal to PMS, are inclined to eat more carbohydrates. For years, the explanation for why giving up smoking and drinking should result in weight gain was dismissively put down to 'comfort eating'. It now seems, however, that the real reason is because ex-smokers and ex-drinkers naturally self-regulate their low mood and counteract withdrawal symptoms by increasing their sugar intake which, in turn, results in weight gain, the liver turning most of the excess carbohydrate into fat. Importantly, this has been confirmed in studies in which animals have shown the same increased appetite for sugar, and accompanying weight gain, following the end of tobacco use. Seasonal affective disorder (SAD) is a syndrome involving recurrent depressions at the same time of the year. It, too, is characterized by carbohydrate cravings which improve mood and lessen fatigue, suggesting that the mind is self-medicating in order to restore the balance. But the precise route by which carbohydrates work to improve mood and energy is still unknown. The most popular explanation is that by stimulating the release of insulin – sometimes known as the hunger hormone – from the pancreas, a high-carbohydrate meal initiates a complex physiological process that results in the increased serotonin production.

Bulimics are an extreme case in point. People with bulimia almost invariably report that bingeing episodes are precipitated by a tense or depressed mood, and that the eating of calorie-rich carbohydrates improves it.

But one needn't go to extremes to prove the point. It has been found that women on a 1000-calorie-a-day diet – the sort usually recommended as being perfectly safe by slimming magazines and organizations – also have lowered levels of serotonergic activity, increasing the pressure on a person to binge when food is available. Dr Hill of the Academic Unit of Psychiatry, Leeds University notes:

> Not only are women more at risk of eating disorders because of the cultural pressures to be thin, but perhaps they are also biologically at risk as a result of the change in neurochemical responsiveness. Dieting appears to be the key which unlocks this important biological consequence.
>
> *Proceedings of the Nutrition Society*

It comes as little surprise, then, that this wilful variation in serotonin levels caused by even mild dieting increases the chances of putting the whole regulatory mechanism out of kilter: dieters are eight times more likely to become bulimics than non-dieters. Anorexics, on the other hand, tend to have higher than normal levels of serotonergic activity, suggesting that for this eating disorder, food deprivation is associated with a good mood.

Whatever the full facts of this relatively new area of research turn out to be, we have yet another means by which dieting makes you fat: by inducing depression, dieting encourages us to eat more carbohydrates, in particular calorie-rich simple carbohydrates or sugars, which lead to mood-elevating chemical changes in the brain.

The message is clear: the biggest favour we can do ourselves – our figure, our health and our good spirits – is to give up dieting and learn to re-adopt a reasonable attitude to food. Only then will our bodies find their best weights.

7

Dieting: Just Another Fact of Life?

Why do I diet? It's irrelevant *why* I go on a diet. Just tell me where to find one that works!

Iris, Oxford

Iris is wrong. One of the single biggest mistakes you can make is to believe that it is 'irrelevant' *why* you are dieting. The absolute golden rule of losing weight is 'never underestimate intangibles': ideas, thoughts, attitudes, words. Looking at those will stand you in far better stead than any amount of calorie counters. If you can understand the reasons why you want to lose weight you may well find that the amount of weight you wish to lose is halved, that your ideal is not a stone away (months in the future) but just a few pounds away, a mere week or two. That means that instead of fretting and starving you can relax and be happy because your goal is so close.

Or, indeed, you may realize that you do not need to lose any weight at all.

We've looked at the big three reasons for dieting: men, clothes and health, but there are scores of others. High among them is the feeling that dieting is just another fact of modern life.

Many of us no longer really think about the shape which suits us best. Faced with a million 'thin women' images, constantly surrounded by diet talk, we simply feel that we too must 'get thinner'. Virtually everybody knows at least one woman who continues dieting even though she has reached a weight at which she looks lovely. How many of us – hellbent on losing weight – actually *listen* to what our partner says about our figure? How many ignore the advice proffered by a girlfriend, even though we would value her judgement on any other subject? And I bet there's not one in a thousand who pays attention to parents ('Oh Mum, always trying to fatten me up . . .'). But the truth is, the people around us are very good judges of what shape suits us, if only we would listen. In researching this book I have heard one particular refrain from partners, parents and friends, young and old. Let Leslie speak for them all:

> My girlfriend simply won't listen to me about her figure. She's lovely as she is, but she's got this fixed idea that she's got to be 'thin' and nothing I say will sway her. Of course it's her body, but – how can I put it? – it's gone beyond reason.

We would all do well to listen to Hannah's experience:

> I wanted to lose weight for ages. It began when I got a new job in London and I had to spend an hour on the train commuting to work each morning and evening. I passed the time by buying magazines. Two hours each day of gazing at pencil-thin beauties began to get to me. I started dieting. It was dreadful – I used to feel sick and faint – but with a constant battle I kept the weight off.
>
> Then, one day, eighteen months later, I came across a batch of photos of me before I lost weight. I thought I looked great. You see I was sufficiently distanced from my old self to see how I really looked. I stopped dieting then and there.

For most of us, it is extremely difficult nowadays to be objective about our bodies. Many women already have a fabulous figure but they cannot see it, and continue the dieting misery for no good reason at all.

One of the first things I noticed when I began this book was that there is a difference between the two questions.

Why do you diet?
and
Why do you want to lose weight?

Why do you diet? invokes this sort of response:

> A hundred reasons. A thousand reasons. The old man. My
> women friends. Doctors. Clothes. But mostly because I'd be
> bored if I wasn't on a diet. What would I talk to the girls
> about at work, for goodness sake?
>
> Joyce, Kent

In other words, dieting has become so much a part of our lives
that we often do it simply because we feel left out if we don't.
Food, weight and calories are among the most important topics
of conversation for many women. Over the years dieting has
turned into a national obsession. When I was at university in the
1970s, I used to eat in the student canteen. One day I was queueing
for a cup of coffee with a male fellow student. 'Sugar?' he asked.
'No thanks,' I replied, never having taken sugar in my coffee.
'Oh,' said he, 'are you on a diet?'
I was vastly insulted because I immediately concluded he
thought I was fat and needed to slim. It worried me for weeks.
Today, in a similar situation, not even the most supersensitive
person would be upset by that remark, because *everybody* – fat and
thin – diets. The other day I was in a bar when a group of eight
young women came in. In their early thirties, they were clearly
intelligent and independent, dressed in an unconventional,
slightly arty way, and, judging by the bottles of wine they ordered,
successful. Not one was overweight. Immediately they sat down
they all started talking about diets and slimming.
Many women go along, year after year on a diet, never really
expecting to lose weight. Perhaps they don't actually need to,
but fear that if they don't diet they will put weight on. Indeed,
some women have a morbid fear of gaining even a few pounds,
as if life would suddenly become terrible for them. At a party in
London recently, Judy, a thin friend, was chatting to me about a
woman we both know, and evaluating her chances of snaffling
a man:
'She's quite attractive. I mean she's *slim* . . . ,' said Judy, in a
tone that said, 'Slimness is the one essential feature of female
attractiveness.'
I burst out laughing at the unwitting criticism of my own figure,
and explained that it is actually possible to be quite *curvy,* or even
rounded, and still be attractive. (Her husband, who had just made

a pass at me, evidently thought so.) There are scores of thin women whose looks I admire, but I do not admire thinness as a thing in itself. Yet many unattractively thin people imagine that all manner of horrors will befall them if they put on flesh.

Liz, a quite thin Oxford accountant, said to me recently of a very thin friend: 'Oh, gosh, don't we all envy Bella her lovely figure.' Her comment sprang not so much from generosity, as from old-fashioned female competitiveness. Well no, I didn't envy Bella her figure, which seemed to me thin without being graceful. But while Liz implied that my figure was not what she admired, I thought it too rude to say to her, 'I dislike both your figures and I would prefer you not to assume that I envy them.' It's all part of an *uncritical* worship of thinness, in which an ungainly thin person is always valued above a comely, curvy figure. We need to learn to admire handsome examples of *all* figures from Jerry Hall to the voluptuous Dawn French. French does not have 'a pretty face in spite of being fat'; her figure is an intrinsic part of her beauty and appeal.

For many, dieting is more a state of mind than an activity, and it's significant that many psychologists prefer to use the term 'restrained eater' instead of 'dieter', and characterize a restrained eater not as a person who deliberately cuts the number of calories she eats, but as one who merely *intends* to cut calories, whether or not she does it in fact. For some it's even a way of life:

> I mean, if I didn't diet, and announced I wasn't going to diet, people would immediately criticize, look for faults so they could pull me apart and say, 'Who the hell do you think you are that you're exempt from dieting like the rest of us? Think yourself so perfect do you?' Dieting has become associated with virtue. It's as if 100 years ago someone said, 'I don't need to have Christian principles.'
>
> Gillian

Two years ago I would sadly, angrily have agreed with this remark. Now my response is: Yes, it's still true, *but it is beginning to change.* When a newspaper printed an unflattering snap of TV presenter Judy Finnegan in a bikini on the beach, women all over England were disgusted, not at Judy's figure, but at the paper: 'She's wonderful, leave her alone, we all look like that sometimes,' was the message. Similarly, many people – male and female – were sickened by the fact that the uproar over the Duchess of York's semi-naked photos was more to do with her supposed 'fatness' than with her relationship with John Bryan:

> It made me furious, people going on about her weight. Her body belongs to her, it's not public property. Who the hell are strangers to pass judgement? I'm not particularly sympathetic to the Duchess personally, but that's another matter altogether.

And, I noticed, it tended to be men who said she was not fat anyway:

> What I've always liked about her is she's a real shape. Not a knobbly fencepost.
>
> Ian, 26

> What's wrong with her figure? It's all right by me! Personally I liked her even larger.
>
> Ben, 59

There is a growing backlash against the stultifying uniformity the fashion for extreme slenderness has imposed upon women. People are beginning, nowadays, to recognize and admire determined non-dieters: or better still, they are admiring *carefree* non-dieters. They may also envy them.

Why Do You Want to Lose Weight?

There are, of course, a score – nay, a million – uncategorizable reasons why women say they want to be thinner, some comic, some tragic. One lady became an obsessive – and very successful – dieter after being stuck for several hours down a pothole on a school expedition, an experience repeated recently in New Zealand when a twenty-nine-year-old public health nurse became trapped in the evocatively named Rumbling Gut Cave in Waitomo. 'It was the first narrow bit. Wide at the top, wide at the end but very small in the middle,' said the potholer. 'I got my head and shoulders through but my bottom wouldn't follow. I couldn't go forward and I couldn't go back.' Luckily, her friends, after trying in vain for two hours, called in the Fire Service who used drills and chisels and finally put a rope around her ankles and pulled so that she shot out like a cork from a bottle. The lady in question, who was a size 18, had joined a gymnasium the day before, intending to shed 25 kg. But the interesting part of the story is that a rescue organizer said that but for her weight she might not have lived: the extra flesh had saved her from dying of hypothermia. Rosalind, on the other hand, was trapped by fire in a bathroom and had to climb through a horribly narrow window:

> I got stuck. I was terrified. My bottom was still inside, about to be roasted like a sausage, and my arms were outside waving around like a pair of cocktail sticks. The firemen were squirting water everywhere. Somehow I popped out. I've been on a diet ever since!

Another woman explained that she had to lose weight in order to reach the drain between the side of her house and her garden fence. This recalls surely one of the most unusual reasons I've come across (perfectly true as I have seen it for myself), namely that the lady in question, Alana, had no choice but to get thin because her new home was one half of an old house which had been divided into two down the middle of the staircase. Unless she went on bread and water rations every few weeks, it was impossible to get upstairs.

Doctors are often telling their patients to lose weight on the promise (usually false, as it turns out) of a whole variety of health benefits: thinness is supposed to be better for your heart, your liver, your left elbow, and your unborn child. One mother inverted the last reason in the following refreshing way:

> My magic diet is called *The Offspring Diet*. The bottom line? Have children. Plenty of them. I was so sick during my pregnancies that even my feet lost weight. Then the kiddies would arrive and start to wear me away. I've calculated it takes about one child per stone (stone and a quarter if you're lucky enough to get a hyperactive specimen). Four children equals four stone. I'm thinking about having a fifth. There's no way I can get into that new dress I bought the other day unless I do.

And here's another gem:

> I met Gary. A real dish. Gorgeous. But there was one prob-
> lem. He was big. Enormous. He played rugby for just about
> every team in London and was the size of a haystack.
> Trouble was, there wasn't enough room in the bed for the
> two of us. I was only a student then and couldn't afford to
> buy another bed, so I had to go on a diet. I lost two stone
> in two months, then I went off Gary and on a skinny little
> fellow who'd never seen a rugger ball in his life, so I put
> everything back on in a fortnight of celebration.

Some women diet for other women:

> I'm seventeen years old, my friends are all slim, I haven't
> so far had trouble with boyfriends. I've been going out with
> good-looking guys steadily since I was fourteen, while a lot
> of girls in my class still have no one. But I do feel left out:
> my clothes aren't so fashionable and my pals are constantly
> teasing me to lose weight.

(Might I suggest that your pals' teasing has more to do with your
enviable success with boys than with your figure?) It is well known
that pressure put on women to diet often comes, not from men,
but from women themselves:

> Funnily enough, I don't mind not looking my best with
> fellas. I'm happily married and all that. But at work there
> are several really cool, sophisticated women (very thin of
> course) and I always feel inferior, which, I suspect, is pre-
> cisely what they want.

I received a letter recently from a woman whose entrepreneurial
father charged £60 for a fortnight's course of milkshake, energy
shakes and vitamins. When his company went bust he blamed his
plump daughter because even she had been unable to stick to the
miserable plan, and had been, therefore, a bad advertisement for
it! Any man who sets up dodgy slimming ventures ought to be
forced to drink his energy shakes until he pops.

Weddings are a big incentive: wedding-dress makers are always
being called in at the last minute to expand the dress, because

most brides overestimate the amount they'll lose before the great day. One lady I read about astonished the seamstresses when she went up two sizes between fittings!

In my experience many of us don't *really* know – beyond a vague sense that life will improve – why we want to lose weight. This is partly because there are so many fallacies surrounding what is popularly termed 'overweight'.

Fallacy: Being 'Overweight' Is Ageing

Studies have shown plump women live longer, age better and don't show wrinkles.

Dr Tom Sanders, nutritionist, King's College, London

Independent on Sunday

Extreme thinness is a much more cruel enemy to beauty than extreme stoutness.

Beauty and How to Keep It, by a Professional Beauty

'After forty,' exclaims Barbara Cartland, 'a woman has to choose between losing her figure or her face. My advice is to keep your face, and stay sitting down.'

A bit sweeping perhaps, and I certainly don't hold with this dim view that women lose whichever way they turn. But, if keeping your figure means keeping the figure of a twenty-year-old, there's something in it. That's not good for your looks. Plumping up a bit as you get older is brilliant for your face *and* your figure. What's more, the menopause occurs several years later in plump women than in lean ones.

Compare that with the Duchess of Windsor's famous comment: 'One can never be too rich or too thin.' (It's always amused me that the Duchess, a dog lover, surrounded herself with those marvels of rotundity – pugs.) Her remark strikes me as possibly the stupidest thing she ever said: extreme wealth has an excellent track record of stifling the soul, making people mean, out of touch and discontented. And with few exceptions excessive thinness does horrors to your appearance sooner or later. But there are two distinct issues here: *being thin* and *getting thin*.

Getting thin – excessive dieting – once past your twenties, is likely to have a bad effect on your face. After all, if the natural ageing process involves the face gradually losing fat under the skin, why hasten it along? Those endless slimming magazine success stories – women who lose huge numbers of stones – do not dwell on the hundreds of women for whom weight loss means a haggard, drooping face, flabby arms and stretch marks. Or on those women who have to have corrective surgery to get rid of excess skin. Many women, lulled by the media hype of slimming, are shocked to find that, having lost a significant amount of weight, they are left looking not only older but rather as if they've been put into a skin boilersuit several sizes too large. Frances:

> I nearly killed myself dieting because I felt unattractive, and quite honestly I've simply swopped one set of problems for another. I was happier as I was. I dieted because 'friends' were constantly on at me about being unhealthy. Now I feel I look five years older.

A Weight Watchers promotional booklet I received recently comprised a selection of 'Before' and 'After' photographs of successful slimmers. A good half of them looked older than before the diet. The fact that they had been featured none the less, suggests one of two things: either Weight Watchers are desperate for successful slimmers, or the current drive for thinness above all else has gone completely barmy.

It is not only crash dieting, but also simply keeping yourself thinner than your natural weight that can be ageing. Many women in their forties are obsessed with maintaining the 'youthful' body they had in their twenties for no better reason than the popular nonsense that it is laudable to have 'kept your girlish figure'. To gain weight gently and moderately as you grow older is now known – medically – to be natural, healthy and youthful. Marie Helvin has spoken openly about being significantly more curvaceous than in her modelling heyday. She's hardly stout, but the fact of having allowed herself to gain weight has no doubt helped her keep her looks so well. A female professor I know in a certain university town, though well over fifty and very ample, has an adoring following of young male undergraduates and is one of the few women about whom one can literally say 'she seems to get younger each time I see her'. There is no doubt that her appeal is (in addition, of course, to her intelligence) closely tied up with her size and physical stature.

115

How well we age has a great deal to do with our genes, over which we have no control. But, after genes come the three Ss: Smoking, Sun and Size. If you want to stay youthful, give up smoking (it not only causes wrinkles round the mouth, but can age by up to ten years the very fabric of your skin), keep well out of the sun, and *plump up a bit.* What is elegant and sleek in one's twenties can easily look gaunt in the thirties and forties and positively scraggy thereafter.

Fallacy: 'Overweight' People Are Unhappy

Thin people are unhappy, Black, white, yellow people are unhappy. Young people are unhappy – oh, and old people. The truth is we're *all* unhappy some of the time. But if you stand out in some way – by being overweight, for example – people notice your unhappiness and remember it. And of course there are all those endless slimming magazines battering us into believing it. Designating groups of people 'unhappy' is too often an insidious way of discriminating against them. I thought I was hearing things the other day when, turning on my radio, I listened to a man declare that if he knew his unborn child was going to be gay he would have it aborted, 'because gay people are unhappy'. It did not seem to have occurred to him that the only reason his child would have been unhappy would have been because of appalling attitudes like his.

Not so very long ago the stereotype was 'fat and jolly', perhaps because, until recently, food and plenty have always been appreciated for the wondrous gifts they are, and not overladen with guilt. As Dr Thomas Short commented in 1727. 'A cheerful temper does much to fatten the body, hence the proverb "Laugh and be fat" is not without its reason and philosophy.' It should therefore come as no surprise that research shows plump people to be more psychologically stable and to commit fewer suicides.

It is also a complete fallacy that a fat person must be fat for some terrible psychological reason – a recent open letter to *Woman* magazine is eloquent on the subject:

I'm not fat because of some dreadful thing that happened

116

to me in the past and from which I'm trying to hide, finding comfort in food.

Also, just for the record, can I make it clear that I wasn't sexually assaulted when I was younger, nor has a man let me down so badly that I'm trying to make myself unattractive so that others won't fancy me in the future.

It is typical of our society's vacuous love of psycho-speak that it should have so widely accepted the silly notion that women put on weight largely as a form of self-defence in a male-dominated world. And, while slimming magazines are always ready to cite horror stories of people who before the miracle weight loss were fat and miserable, they never seem to make the connection that the misery is largely induced by publications such as theirs. As for the minority of people who are fat, and unhappy because of it, we all have it within our power to prevent this. Make sure you are never one of those 'well-meaning' people who oh so kindly offer suggestions on how to slim. We can all be happy with our size – whatever it is – if only other people will let us.

Fallacy: 'Overweight' People Are Greedy

Twelve out of thirteen studies reviewed in *The Energy Balance and Obesity in Man* found the intake of heavier people less than or equal to that of thin people.

Susan Kano, *Never Diet Again*

This is a favourite area of research for the eager nutritionist. It's like one of those happy card tricks that baffle the intuition and wow your friends. 'Do you want to see something strange?' says the researcher to his new student. 'Then do a study on how much skinny people eat as compared to large ones.' Time and time again these studies come up with the same conclusion. They both, on average, eat about the same amount.

This doesn't mean that people don't get fat by eating too much, it just means that the quantity you eat is not the only factor involved. Metabolism differs. One person can have a metabolism that's up to twice as efficient as another person's: in other words she needs half as much food to do the same job. Feed these two people the same meal, and the first will end up storing much

117

more as fat than the second. The veteran nutritionist Dr Elsie Widdowson, who began researching the problem during the war when rationing was inevitable, commented in *The Times*:

> What came out was the enormous variation in energy intake, in every age group. In each group there were some people eating twice as many calories as others. It wasn't because they were greedy, or fat. Why was a bit of a mystery, and nobody's got to the bottom of it even today.

It also seems likely that some people, for genetic reasons, are more likely than others to store energy as fat. In this case, it is not a matter of being overweight, but rather of being at the weight to which your genes incline you. Although even genes are not wholly reliable, for, out of a family of super-skinnies, I am the only one endowed with the magical gift of putting on weight by simply looking at a doughnut.

For a while, researchers thought heaviness might also be to do with the fact that thin people eat more slowly and more regularly than fat people. But this was also disproved. It turned out that poor eating behaviour was the result of the psychological effects of dieting, not the cause of weight gain. Behaviour programmes which teach large people to 'eat like thin people' are therefore based on another fallacy.

Fallacy: Dieting Displays Willpower

Abstainer, n. A weak person who yields to the temptation of denying himself a pleasure.
> Ambrose Bierce, *The Devil's Dictionary*

Willpower is usually seen as an essential *part* of the process of slimming, rather than an end in itself. But for some women willpower – the idea of rigid control – is the mainspring of their dieting. Diets are difficult. It is easy to fail them. It is also ignominious to fail them (dieters are constantly being harangued as weak-willed, self-indulgent, greedy). The successful dieter succeeds not only by virtue of losing weight, but also because she has displayed an enviable resolution. She has distinguished herself by her fortitude: denial is a virtue. In Jeneffer Shute's powerful novel, *Life-*

Size, about an anorexic, the triumphant sense of having had the willpower to starve herself so thin and to resist temptation motivates the heroine.

For non-anorexic women willpower is a more insidious feature of dieting than they may be aware. When diets fail, the dieter blames herself, rather than the diet. And since 95 per cent of diets fail, for many women the relationship with food is one of endless cycles of guilt and denial, guilt and denial, guilt and denial. Doctors too often use willpower as a stick with which to beat their (supposedly) overweight patients. Janet, a GP who phoned me one day from her holiday cottage in Ireland, was particularly angry about precisely this point:

> It breaks my heart to say it, but GPs are notoriously stupid in their appeals to willpower. Never mind that in many cases heavier women eat no more calories than skinny ones and often many fewer, that dieting fails for 95 women out of 100, that every woman has her own natural weight and that it is wicked and unhealthy to encourage her to adopt a thinner one simply because that happens to be the current fashion. In short, willpower has little to do with it. It is nevertheless a very rare GP who does not make tiresome and erronous appeals to willpower.
>
> (My paraphrase)

So, stop worrying about it. Virtually every woman you pass on the street will have discovered, like you, that diets don't work in the long term (and not even, very often, in the short term). Even laboratory animals fail diets. It's the bodily instinct. As soon as calorie restriction is over, rats go straight back to their previous weight. They don't start stuffing the moment they go off a diet, they just eat normally and return to their normal weight. It's the natural thing to do. Willing yourself to remain skinny when you're naturally large is an unnatural thing to do.

Now let's look at this willpower business the other way round. I would have said that often successful dieting reveals a weak will, not a strong one. A person who diets may be a person who hasn't the courage to be individual. Someone who takes one look at a supermodel picture and loses all self-respect. Most women who diet do not need to lose weight, but a weak will dupes them into believing that just a few pounds more and it'll be wake-up-as-

119

Cindy-Crawford-in-the-morning time. Even according to the latest government figures, only a small percentage of women are 'obese': yet 90 per cent of women go on diets. On the other hand there is everything to admire about the woman who has the strength to resist the pressure. For such a woman, we are talking true willpower, because the pressures of fashion are very, very great.

Fallacy: I Diet For Myself

Why do you diet?
I diet to lose weight.
Why do you want to lose weight?
I want to lose weight – for myself. To please myself.
You go through all the misery and frustration to please yourself?
(Pause). I'll feel healthier and happier when I've lost weight.
You seem to me healthy and happy now.
Yes – but . . .
So, you subject yourself year upon year, decade upon decade, to frustrating and unsuccessful regimes, on the off-chance that if it works you might feel healthier and happier?
It must work someday.

This imaginary conversation might apply to a score of people I know, several millions I don't know, and myself. Never, in the whole of my life, can I *honestly* say that I dieted for me alone. I've dieted because of peer pressure; I've dieted for men; I've dieted so that I won't have to walk out of the shop when I discover that their size 14 is 'cut rather small'; I've dieted because my doctor prods my tummy; but, most pernicious of all, my motivation is always partly to do with how I'll appear to the vast impersonal world. This last is what I call the S-Factor. My friend Sally, who invented the term, describes it like this:

The S-Factor is the Stranger Factor. It's the power of the stranger in the street. I want to be able to walk down the street and not have that person think that I'm over-weight. That's all. If fashion changes and the stranger on the street, male or female, starts to admire bigger women, then I'll worry less. I know it's weak of me and I ought not

120

to care. I know I ought to have more self-esteem, but I don't. For me the S-Factor is all important. It's the true scale of approval. If you pass on the S-Factor, then you pass as a woman, and to hell with what your friends say.

You might also call it the Street-Factor, the Social-Factor, even the Subliminal-Factor. It's that feeling, that niggling concern which never quite goes away, that, irrespective of whether or not people make comments or look at you, there is at least a quiet consensus of opinion among those whom you pass, which is either in your favour or against you. In truth, most of them don't even notice you, and, if they do, probably don't think anything about it: they're too busy worrying what you will think of them. But part of you believes they do. And that is enough to make you fret.

The S-factor, in other words, is the means by which cultural pressure works. When we look in a magazine, see a film, read an advertisement – it all creates an impression. If every time we see a beautiful woman she's as thin as a rake, it's not surprising that pretty soon we're going to feel that only by being thin can we get the world's approval. Constantly the media message is 'Look! This is what the people out there think is admirable. Are you like that?'

The recent swing towards a Seventies' fashion revival is a wonderful example of cultural pressure and the S-Factor at work. I have yet to meet anybody who doesn't agree that Seventies' clothes are pretty hideous: those clodhopping shoes, flapping flares and skimpy lace vests. Yet suddenly, in 1993, women's magazines and fashion shows – without consulting us, the consumers – announced that Seventies' fashion was in. Sure enough, the shops are stocked with the stuff. Did they do it as a joke, to see if they could get away with such an absurdity? First, the fashion victims change their wardrobes. Next, the fashion-victims' friends started making little Seventies purchases: not the flares, perhaps, but a clodhopper or two at forty quid. Eventually, after months of constant Seventies' fashion images, we will be battered into thinking 'Perhaps they're not *quite* as hideous as I first thought...' and, exhausted, will give in. By which time it'll be on to Twenties' fashions...

As it is with clothes, so it is with figures: with the irritating difference that figures, instead of hopping gaily from decade to decade (if only 1890s figures would become fashionable), just go on getting thinner. Only in very few cases can anybody really claim that their desire to diet is not brought about to large extent by cultural pressure. If, by some miracle, skinny fashions change and suddenly all the beautiful models weigh not 8 st but 13 st, then of course people will start claiming the reason they're eating eight Big Macs a day is because it makes them feel healthier and happier to do so. It's instructive to remember that at the end of the last century pills called 'Wateon' used to sell like hot cakes. As Jo angrily remarks:

> My doctor thinks I ought to lose weight because I'll feel better when I'm thinner, even though I feel great now. My husband thought I ought to lose weight because he's worried what his friends will think. The mags say I ought to lose weight because thin is in. My mother says I ought to lose weight because it shows self-control. The clothes shop insists I lose weight because otherwise I can't buy anything half decent. How can I help thinking that everybody else out there is secretly thinking I'm too fat and I should lose weight? And then I think to myself, hey, where in the hell do *my* wishes come into all this?

The strength of the S-Factor can be considerable, even if it concerns only one stranger. Recently, there was an interesting experiment in which various people selected at random were invited to take part in a 'nutritional exercise'. The volunteers duly gathered: they were instructed to proceed through room A and out again to reach room B, the laboratory. Here they would be able to choose their food – a good selection, they were cheerily assured. In room A was a young and beautiful model, deliberately put there by the researchers for this experiment but apparently engaged in some completely different research as far as the volunteers knew. The researchers discovered that the sort of food people chose in the laboratory, room B, depended heavily on the sort of food the model was eating in the intermediate room A. She was eating a salad and lean chicken breast? Salad and lean chicken breast was what people picked up in the lab. She was having an enormous bag of fish and chips? An enormous bag of fish and chips became the most popular dish for that day. When the model ate fruit salad, fruit salad was in demand: and when she ate chocolate gâteau with a monument of whipped cream on top, that was the dessert of choice. No one cottoned on. But the point made was dramatic and obvious. We are all very easily influenced by what people around us do and seem to approve of, especially if they happen to be beautiful.

So, if our minds are such that we can be encouraged subconsciously to alter our choice of meals just by passing an eating model, is it any wonder that we are obsessed with slenderness and dieting, even when often our bodies are most comfortable, and probably more healthy, as we are? We live and breathe dieting. Virtually everything in our culture is sold with a bit of help from thinness, including improbables such as cars, insurance, even lavatory cleaners. And also, as Carrie points out, rich fatty foods:

> On telly it's always a thin woman who's scoffing cream buns and indulging in a bit of 'naughty but nice'. She's usually got blonde hair, lots of lipstick and not very much on her legs. You never see a picture of a fat woman on the billboards eating. It's the thin one again who's piling calories on to her plate, her lipstick miraculously unsmudged and the legs still showing. I pick up a magazine, and what do I see? She's at it again! Gobble, gobble, gobble.

I know plenty of fit, radiant women who have wonderful, happy jobs and lovely, stable relationships and perfect health; yet, because they're a stone above what they imagine they ought to be, they're constantly perturbed by diets. Their size gives them presence in the office or the boardroom and their blokes say they love a woman who looks like a woman. Their vitality and enthusiasm tells them their body is in wonderful health. Yet their minds keep nagging that they'd be better off if they were skinny. They worry that their partner is biased, their friends are just being nice, and that their success would be better appreciated. It's nonsense. They know it's nonsense. They know that they're at their natural weight and every bit of common sense says they ought to stay that way, but still they buy any magazine with 'Revolutionary New Diet' scribbled on the cover, are blushingly coy about their exact poundage, and always purchase foods with 'lite' in the name. I was one of them.

Of course, the S-Factor is not limited to women. Men are influenced by it, too. As Sally's husband says with a chortle:

> When I was younger I really used to worry about the size of

my shoulders. I got it fixed into my head that a real man has these huge great wings extending from his neck with muscly arms dangling from the ends. I did circuit training, weightlifting, ate body-building foods and joined a rugby club. For years I behaved like a complete idiot and now here I am, with these enormous shoulders. And what good has it done me? Nowt. Sally tells me that the one thing that put her off when we first met was my big shoulders.

The S-Factor is intrinsic to human behaviour. We are a social species – one important reason why we are so successful and now (alas) dominate the earth. Part of being a social species means that each of us cares, to some degree, what the rest of the world thinks. This has its good side as well as its bad. Without the S-Factor, people wouldn't give a damn. Our streets would be filled with colourful, well-balanced people wearing everything and nothing of all sizes, not caring a penny what other people think about them, and succumbing to every unreasonable whim and misdemeanour imaginable.

But the S-factor can get dangerously out of hand. Cultural pressure can kill. As everyone knows, the rate of occurrence of anorexia is rocketing. Some researchers estimate that up to 20 per cent of women in American suffer to some degree. Of those, roughly 20 per cent will die from it. Now read this:

Anorexia is, on average, ten and a half times more common in women than in men.

For a long time nobody could really understand why this should be the case. Various theories were thrown about. But, recently, the chilling answer has become much clearer. Do you know how many more advertisements and articles promoting weight loss women's magazines carry than men's?

Ten and a half times more.

One of the techniques used in the treatment of anorexia is to present women with a photograph of themselves in an attempt to make them see that they are too thin. Yet, at the same time as doctors use pictures of anorexics to get people to eat, advertisements and magazine photos use pictures of borderline anorexics to get people to diet.

I am not, nor have I ever been, anorexic, but clearly the disorder provides a striking example of the S-Factor out of control. The heroine of *Life-Size* is severely anorexic. When her doctors, friends and relatives tell her she is far too thin and looks dreadful that way, she thinks them either envious or ignorant. She is appealing to some higher aesthetic authority, the authority of the S-Factor.

So, when you consider your reasons for dieting, *really* think about where they are coming from. If you find that you diet for no better reason than to please a bunch of strangers, *STOP.* Life is too precious to waste on them.

8

The Untold Story

I'm a size 18. And I'm happy. I love my body. My man loves my body. The only time I've ever been unhappy was when I went on a 1000-calories-a day diet and nearly ruined my life. The size 14 years were the worst years of my life.

Bernice, Loughborough

So I'm supposed to be miserable am I? Fifteen stone of misery, eh? Let me tell you something, Weight Watchers: wake up! Anyone who gets conned into thinking the world gets rosy only when you're thin as a bicycle pump is too stupid to be happy.

Jane, Exeter

Show me a dieter and I'll show you unhappiness.

Mrs G.J., London

Slimming magazines are stuffed with success stories. Ordinary women's magazines, when copy is short, usually manage to dredge up a character who's lost an unbelievable number of stone, and pose her standing skinny in her old clothes and looking comically into the yawning gap between new waistline and old. Next to the photos is a lengthy article about how her weight used to shoot up and up between unsuccessful diets, until suddenly a wedding, or perhaps the catty remark of a neighbour, gave her resolution, and bingo! here she is, a new woman.

Yawn, yawn, yawn. These stories are monotonously the same – how terrible life was before the diet, how wonderful life is since the diet.

This is the story that is told. I am not for one moment undermining the women in these scenarios, or their amazing achievements. Of course there are people who are overweight and miserable and whose lives do indeed seem to start afresh after successful weight loss. The people I am criticizing are those who advertise such stories. They give only one small part of the truth, and these articles are used to batter other women into believing that if they would lose weight, they too would be happy. As it says in a current advertisement for Rosemary Conley Diet and Fitness clubs, 'You can join the millions who have successfully reshaped their bodies and their lives'. What the slimming clubs and magazines don't tell you is the subject of this chapter: the *untold* story.

To Hell With Diets!

In October 1993 *Woman* magazine published a letter of mine announcing that I was writing this book and requesting any stories, tips, anecdotes or information concerning slimming. I also asked to hear from women who were size 14+ and proud of it. I have quoted three, above. Here are three more from the scores I received:

> I am size 20 and not on any diet at all! I take plenty of exercise and I live a very full and active life. I dress well. I have a boyfriend and several other admirers! . . . I feel so sorry for the girls I see who deny their size by cutting labels out, squeezing into clothes too small and saying they are much slimmer than they are. I tell people I'm a size 20 and very happy too.
>
> V.S., London

> I'm 13 st and 5ft 9ins. That's not very big, but it's big enough for me to have wasted a good portion of my life on diets. Then I stopped. I've never been happy at any other weight, and no matter what I do I always end up coming back to this one. So why be a patsy to fashion? Every woman has a natural size that suits her best. Women who don't let their bodies be as they want to be will always be unhappy.
>
> Natalie, Derbyshire

> Two things have made me unhappy in my life. My divorce

and dieting. It's no coincidence that my marriage went to pieces when I was making the hardest effort to lose weight. The good news is that now I've given up dieting and am back to weighing 14 st 6 lbs my ex-husband and I are falling in love again. Happy, happy, happy!

J.J., Bristol

Why did I get so many replies? Quite simply, because there are so many women who are happy the way they are naturally, but whose lives have been made unhappy – sometimes appallingly unhappy – by the constant insistence that all women should be a size 12 or below. Many of the correspondents had been through the miseries of trying to diet, and emerged triumphantly anti-dieting. Why, then, do we never read about these positive women? Why are we only ever told how miserable they are?

The most important reason is: *because nobody profits by them.* Indeed, when the pressure on women to be thin, thin, thin abates, an awful lot of people stand to lose an awful lot of money. The dieting industry is worth billions. Nearly 50 per cent of British women are size 16+. There's a lot of cash to be made out of haranguing them into believing that health and happiness depend on skinniness. But it does not stop there. In 1988, *Cosmopolitan* discovered that 78 per cent of its readers wanted to lose weight, even though most were already at the 'recommended' weight – findings confirmed by the academic journals. Most women want to be *below* average weight – they want to be unnaturally thin. So they buy diet products.

But from the entrepreneur's point of view it gets better still. Diet products don't work. Time after time it has been shown that 95 per cent, even up to 98 per cent of diets don't work, and when they fail the dieter blames herself, not the product. So, instead of realizing that the products' claims were utterly unreasonable, we have a good old binge to get ourselves nice and ready for the next round, then trip out and buy a whole set more diet products. The endless miracle success stories featured in magazines and diet books make sure you jolly well keep purchasing the books, videos, pills, powders, potions, exercycles, vitamin supplements, diet drinks, low-fat spreads/yoghurts/cheeses/ice creams (yes, ice creams!), body toners, bodyshapers, body wraps, laxatives, leotards, instant meals, training shoes, steps, rowers, multigyms, weekends for two at the health farm, and, of course, the magazines themselves, which rely so heavily on slimming-related advertisements. The diet industry is an example of economic perpetual motion. It's a gold mine.

Of course, these miracle stories are not just about how nice it is to be a size 10, they're also about how horrible it is to be anything else. Whatever your state of mind, they somehow contrive to suggest that you are unhappy. When Rosemary Conley in *The Hip and Thigh Diet* prints a photograph of her before-I-went-on-a-diet thighs and calls them 'revolting', she knows exactly what she's doing. The word 'revolting' is completely unnecessary – we can have our own thoughts about her legs. She shows them to you and calls them 'revolting' so that you might see *your* thighs (which may well be larger than hers) as 'revolting'. We are not born with such self-disgust, we get it from images like these. Another writer (an eat-raw-foods-until-you-turn-into-a-rabbit evangelist) announces in her first chapter: 'Most of us who are or have ever been overweight have a sense that to some extent we are missing out. We are not as alive as we could be, nor as beautiful, nor as joyous – and we know it.' Rather subtle, this. She starts by niggling. All those gentle qualifiers of the first sentence. That innocent-as-pie development. Then the second sentence contains the stab. Don't kid yourself, she's saying, I *know* you're not happy.

Who is this woman to tell me what I'm not? What does she know about it? That's for me to decide. Keep your moralizing to yourself, madam.

Whatever grandiose claims these miracle diets make, the fact is that their thinly disguised taunts do a great deal more harm than good. Rebecca:

> My husband loves my legs – yes, they're quite chubby but it doesn't bother him. It only started to bother me after I started reading diet books. I was so comfortable with him before and now I'm nervous.

Louise tells an even sadder story:

> My boyfriend didn't even know cellulite was anything out of the ordinary [which, since 80 per cent of women have it, it isn't] until he picked up a slimming book. OK, he's easily influenced, but who isn't these days? Now he keeps suggest-

ing I go to a clinic and have that terrible electric needle treatment.

If writers and diet promoters are so concerned with our happiness, the best way is not to harass us into regimes that will not work. Only then will those who seriously wish to lose weight have a chance of actually succeeding.

For all the sweeping diet claims, a miserable 5 per cent of dieters manage to keep their weight off permanently ('permanently' is deemed to be five years). Some researchers estimate the success rate to be as low as 2 per cent. So next time you are shamed by those miracle success stories, remember the 95 per cent who didn't make it.

But Famous People Are Always Thin

Well, some of them are. Some of the time.

Reading the newspapers and magazines it does sometimes seem as though ordinary women are the only ones with weight problems. Nothing could be further from the truth. To take a sample at random: Melanie Griffith's weight over the last ten years has skittled around from 7 st (dangerously low for a woman of 5 ft 9 ins) up to 13 st. Kathleen Turner, the Duchess of York and Cybill Shepherd all also hit 13 st. Kim Wilde, at 5 ft 5 ins, went up to over 11 st, Belinda Carlisle, at 5 ft 4 ins to over 12 st, and Margot Hemingway outdid the lot of them by topping 15 st. These slimmers suffer weight problems just like the rest of us. The difference is, they tend to do it in secret: their careers depend on staying thin. When their weight shoots up (often as a result of drink and drugs) their publicity agent threatens them with a machine-gun to stay well out of sight. On the rare occasions when they're photographed, they're well camouflaged.

Lean, svelte Faye Dunaway has spoken openly about her eating disorders and how, as a compulsive overeater, she used to hide food all around her house and binge on boxes of biscuits. Nobody who saw her in *Bonnie and Clyde* would have guessed the miseries she went through in order to lose the necessary 20 lbs. She still regularly attends a very strict counselling service for overeaters. Beautiful, talented Judy Garland was almost destroyed by complications arising from her weight problems. Singer Karen Carpenter starved to death at thirty-two years old. Liz Taylor, a celebrated yo-

yo dieter, even published her own diet book after losing vast amounts. Two years later she was back at 13 st. (What is it about the unlucky 13 st? It's my heaviest weight as well.)

The woman who takes my fancy is Kirstie Alley, star of the American soap *Cheers!*. She is 5 ft 7 ins and has fluctuated between 8 st and (guess what) nearly 13 st. I have pictures of her large and small: small, she is indistinguishable from any one of a hundred fashion model types. Large, she is quite magnificent: not only twice as beautiful, but she looks like Kirstie Alley and nobody else.

Perhaps the most public weight battle of all is that of Oprah Winfrey, 5 ft 4 ins and at one time over 15 st. What a sad sign of the times, that she, one of the most successful women in the United States, admits:

> Losing weight was the single greatest accomplishment of my life. Owning my own show, buying a studio, having the number-one talk show in the world, was nothing compared to getting the weight off me. I was a food junkie.

Having at one time got down to 9 st 4 lbs, she then put much of it back on again . . . Then she had the courage to say *ENOUGH IS ENOUGH*, give up dieting and become fit enough to take part in a half-marathon. As she admitted:

> I am a foodaholic. I love eating. I became depressed when I was on a diet. I was starving myself to death. I was finding it hard to think about anything, or anyone, except food. *Then I realized happiness didn't depend on the size of my thighs.*
>
> (My italics)

At the time of writing I believe she has, alas, succumbed to pressures and got thin again . . .

As well as the very famous there are several thousand not-quite-famous women whose lives are a lot less smooth and effortless than they appear: jet-set women who are always slender, immaculately dressed and clutching a glass of champagne and a French cigarette. A society doctor who agreed to speak to me in confidence, commented:

> Eating disorders among such women are almost common-place – and never officially diagnosed. I know many such

131

women, for whom maintaining their svelte figure rules their lives. Of course, they probably would argue it was worth it, since a svelte figure is the most important thing in their life.

One actress whom I know considers any woman over size 10 to be as unfortunate as a hunchback, and yet is too caught up in the endless cycle of trying to look 'perfect' ever to see that life holds more than day after day of saunas, massages, keep-fit sessions, face packs, exercises and rigid, steely food control. Unlike fashion models, she has no professional reason for such behaviour. Indeed, she often complains of being cast only as bimbos! She reminds me of the woman quoted by Shelley Bovey in *Being Fat Is Not a Sin*, who was

> obsessive about her (normal) weight and who has to attend a large number of professional lunches and dinners. Did she know of women who vomited up their meals to prevent weight gain . . .? Did *she* do it? Of course, she said, seeming rather surprised at my question. Doesn't everyone?

So . . . if you feel you are overweight, are you going to battle with yourself until you succeed, then flaunt it to the world to prove a point – or show that you have the courage not to diet, and a great number of better things to do with your time?

Disappointments

Feeling that one is overweight can assume such gigantic proportions in our minds that we quickly come to see the time when we are slim as the beginning of a new life – a life when everything will be wonderful, all our problems solved. I've lost count of how many times I've felt that way myself, in spite of the well-documented disappointment experienced by many successful slimmers. I simply did not believe there was such a thing. How could there be? I just *knew* my life would be transformed. It must be something invented to console fatties.

I lost the weight. On a holiday in Greece I spent each day walking and swimming as if my life depended on it. Each evening I tucked into a hearty meal of lamb kebabs, moussaka, taramasalata, baklava, or whatever, and then went straight to the restaurant lavatory and vomited it up.

When I returned home I was a stone and a half thinner and could fit into all sorts of new clothes. One of my clearest visions is of standing in front of a mirror in Marks & Spencers where I was trying on some shoes. I caught sight of these thin, unrecognizable legs. That was very nice. But, I soon found, that was all. Nothing else had changed. Nobody treated me any differently (except one person who – quite kindly – expressed concern over my gaunt face). My work went on as normal. The pleasure of smaller clothes wore off very quickly, and it was a battle to stop vomiting. Altogether very unpleasant. Within a month or two I put the weight on again.

Rebecca, happily married to Peter, is 5 ft 7 ins and a size 16. She's chatty, energetic and cheerful, and the only time when she wasn't was after going on a crash diet:

> However nice the garments, on me they always looked just short of elegant. I reckoned 1½ st would do the trick. I dieted – lost the weight – but what I hadn't bargained for is that now, in bed with my husband, I felt unsexy. You know the French expression 'A woman should look thin and feel fat'. Before, though I was not happy clothed, I was so proud of my rather curvy figure naked. I used to love to prance about the room feeling utterly sexy getting ready for bed with my husband. After I dieted, I lost that pleasure. For one thing the weight went first off my breasts. But altogether, all over, I felt less desirable. I had to make a choice. I decided to forget being fussy about clothes. I looked OK.
>
> All in all, I'm glad I put the weight back on.

We have already seen how for some women it takes getting thin to make them realize that they weren't fat in the first place. Suzanne had another experience:

> I found myself degenerating into a more superficial person, the more obsessed I became with dieting. It began with the diet itself, but then I was not satisfied without a manicure, without a full make-up. I was having expensive facials once a week, and still I wasn't happy. I got to the stage when I

didn't know when to stop. The time I used to spend reading, visiting friends, doing interesting things, I'd spend elaborately waxing my legs. I became an absolute pain.

The most outrageous thing I heard was from Liz, in Cardiff:

My husband encouraged me to lose weight. When I succeeded he said he preferred me before! I was furious. I demanded why, and after a long hard night of recriminations, he admitted (1) that I was more sexy before – he'd gone for the bimbo image because he thought it would boost *his* image, and (2) that I was 'like every woman – not you any longer'.

Nora:

I once read a shrewd comment by a writer, something like this: 'I am so glad I went to Oxford because if I had not gone I would have such a tremendous respect for anyone who had been there. As it is, I don't care a damn.' That's me and dieting. Before I'd ever been thin I imagined it to be the most holy state. Now that I've been there (5 ft 3 in and 7 st 7 lbs) I don't give a toot. I know what it's like and I'm not particularly impressed. I let my weight go where it takes me.

Having questioned a substantial cross-section of women who had lost weight and were *not* ecstatic about the results, perhaps the most remarkable revelation was that for many of them the standard of men they attracted plummeted. Susan:

I was absolutely convinced that if I lost weight I would be more attractive to men (although admittedly I hadn't had a great deal of trouble before), and if you're simply talking *numbers* that's probably true. I get stared at in the street quite a bit. Men wolf-whistle from building sites. But quite honestly, so what? I realize now I don't need that kind of boost – it's not *me* they're attracted to, it's something quite impersonal. I've grown to hate that kind of intimacy – some creep on a building site leering.

Louise has a similar angle:

When I was larger, I was me, absolutely me alone and nobody else. If a man chatted me up, I knew it was because of me personally. Since I lost weight and began to look more like the magazine ideal, I feel my body comes first. Of course, it's nice to attract men immediately, but that kind of physical attraction can be very superficial. They're thinking about bed – a conquest – half the time, whereas when I was larger I had the impression that men who chatted me up were not so single-minded.

Laura:

Since losing weight, I've had more creeps after me than I ever knew existed before!

Sian:

Some men are so susceptible to peer pressure and their image. A man who goes for a woman who is outside the magazine ideal strikes me immediately as someone who is interesting and self-confident. You've really got to work at sorting out the dross when you're slim.

Rosalind, from Norwich:

I once read a statistic which said that men with larger partners were more likely to have a stable marriage. At first I thought 'how odd', but when you think about it, it's obvious. The man isn't only choosing a woman to boost his image. Look at models and film stars. They have the most disastrous marriage statistics in the world.

As Amber from Glasgow neatly put it:

The man who is impressed by your 34–22–34 figure before yourself, your personality, is likely to be impressed by other women's 34–22–34.

Let some more women speak of their experiences:

I've been on every diet there is. I've had diet pills, laxatives, water pills, even speed. I've also had liposuction. Let me tell

you something. It's all horrible and useless! The only way
to lose weight is to stop worrying about food and learn to
live life pleasantly. That way your body will do what's best
for it.

Jane

So size 14 is big? That's small to us Northerners! I've always
been 'buxom' and now I'm disabled I'm, yes, fat. Size 20/
22 but whilst not proud of it, I'm happy, I survived two
major operations, I appreciate life and the important things,
i.e. relationships, gardening, conversation, humour, etc.
Don't show me a diet . . .

Mavis

I am size 16/18 and I am totally happy that way. I have
been anorexic, have been a compulsive eater and now enjoy
what I call my fat and happy state. No size 10 figure would
ever entice me to go through it again, I'll stay fat thank you.

Carol

The unequivocally large comedian Jo Brand, when asked if she
would take a pill that promised to make her thin, responded: 'Yes,
but only so that I could eat more than I do already.' Then, in
more serious vein, she went on to say: 'If I wasn't fat I wouldn't
feel the way I feel and I wouldn't have the personality I have,
which is all tied up with what it's like to be different from thin
people . . .' She's been through all the dieting nonsense, leading
of course to inexorable weight gain. She now quite rightly points
out that there are a great many more interesting things to do and
think about.

Stories like these abound, it's just that you rarely get a chance
to read them. And it's not only women who diet. According to a
recent Mori survey, one in three men are trying to lose weight.
The difference is, they do it in secret. Many men find the idea of
dieting 'sissy' or unmasculine. But the media is getting to them,
too. The delectable Oscar Wilde is famed for having declared: 'I
can resist anything except temptation'. Today, Norman Schwarz-
kopf, who weighs in at $17\frac{1}{2}$ st, announces: 'I'm on a diet all the
time – except when I'm eating'.

Perhaps the most surprising thing researching this book has
taught me is that, on balance, it is the slim women who suffer

more from the pressures of the thin fashion ideal than larger women. Probably because they have a most unrealistic dread of what life would be like if they put on a few pounds. Curvies, on the other hand, though they may like the idea of losing weight, know full well that life can be blissfully happy whatever size you are. Over the past decade and a half I have been, at different times, both quite thin and quite fat, and I can honestly say that, essentially, nothing in my life changed in either state.

So, even if you are still unhappy with your weight (I know I would prefer mine not to go up again), why not have realistic expectations of how much you need to lose? Don't put your health at risk by aiming for a figure that is very very thin. Most important, don't hide away and put your life on hold until that mythical moment when you are thin. As Rita from Southampton says:

> You're on this earth only once. Don't waste it dieting. Stop dieting and your weight will find its own best place. Stop dieting and be happy!

Part Two

WHAT ARE THE OPTIONS FOR LOSING WEIGHT?

9

The Dieter's Digest

A Summary and Comparison of the Main Non-Surgical Dieting Methods, with Curious Notes

> Sir, I have followed your prescription as if my life depended on it, and have ascertained that during this month I have lost three pounds or a little more. But in order to reach this result I have been obliged to do such violence to all my tastes and all my habits – in a word I have suffered so much – that while giving you my best thanks for your kind directions, I renounce any advantages from them and throw myself for the future entirely into the hands of providence.
>
> Dieter, writing to his doctor in 1925, Quoted in Astwell.

Addicted to buying diet books? Me, too. Until quite recently my fingers would get itchy at the beginning of each year when the new crop of publications hit the shops, and women's magazines teemed with interviews with the super-skinny authors confidentially declaring that before they discovered their plan, life was a humiliating, flab-ruled misery.

I'm just about able to resist them nowadays – and if you read this chapter you'll see why. But even for those of you who are determined not to break the diet-book-buying habit, at least you'd better know what you're addicted to.

In the good old days of the Sixties and Seventies when slimming was really beginning to boom, there was usually one Big One – *The Scarsdale Diet*, Audrey Eyton's *F-Plan* and the like – plus a reasonable crop of others that one could toy with as a backup. But things have changed. Drop down to your local bookshop and

141

you will see that *everybody* is jumping on to the slimming-book bandwagon; doctors, cookery writers, film stars, TV personalities, cranks, complete nonentities. And yes, if you add me, even sex-book writers.

When I began researching this chapter I fully intended to have a complete catalogue of all available diet books, and I duly hurried out to purchase them. However, it quickly became clear that a) such were the numbers of diet books that in doing so I risked bankruptcy; b) if I attempted to outline even a fraction of these often boring, repetitive publications my readers would soon be deeply asleep; and c) titles come and go with such lightning speed that they get out of date before you can say 'cream doughnut'. So in what follows I will be showing how *you* can evaluate the latest diet book for yourself. How you can see through the hype and understand what you are really getting for your money.

First, can you guess how many known methods for weight control there are on record in Britain and America?

Fifty? One hundred? Maybe even 1000?

Answer: well over 30,000.

30,000 methods!

That's a different technique every day of your life from birth until you're eighty-two years old (although if you're planning on lasting that long your best chance is to *give up* buying diet books). Furthermore, I got the 30,000 statistic from a book published in the Eighties. The figure's probably more like 40,000 by now. And that's not including the further umpteen thousand personalized variations and novel regimens invented by you and me and cranky 'doctors' who never publish. Then, of course, there are untold thousands more plans being proposed in other parts of the world – the Austrians, for example, swear by toast crumbs and water, and assiduously put themselves on such a cure several times a year.

Those firmly addicted to weight loss could begin the week with a bit of vertical stomach stapling; spend Tuesday eating only well-cooked bananas; on Wednesday you might give Dr Gordan's Elegant Pills a try; Thursday, you'll probably have to spend in hospital because the stomach staples have ruptured, so while you're there why not have a Garren-Edwards 250cc gastric balloon inserted instead; it's Friday, and since you'll be feeling a bit off colour I suggest you try tuning in to your digestive plane with the aid of an appropriate crystal; Saturday, roll yourself up in muddy rags, and on Sunday round off the week with Dr Long's revolutionary plan, using the unconscious to vibrate away your unwanted adipose deposits. First, take a sip of water, and then recite, eyes closed, the following:

> As the organs of assimilation and elimination are now properly performing their respective duties, the blood is circulating normally, all waste is being carried away and my weight is decreasing. I am growing lighter and lighter each day. Each week, I shall lose two pounds. My food is assimilating properly, all waste is being carried off and I am growing better in every way.

Didn't do the trick? Never mind – keep trying. You have to pick a winner one day.

History is full of weight-loss remedies. But although they have been around for several thousand years, they have only very recently been aimed at women. Most diets throughout history have been designed for vastly wealthy male fatties who had spent their fortunes on eating too many dishes of quails' eggs and honeyed truffles. The work of the Greek doctor Galen (AD 129–199) remained the medical standard for an incredible 1300 years after his death. He announced that he could make any 'sufficiently stout patient moderately thin' by forcing him to run like the blazes, then wiping away the perspiration (which was supposed to contain fat) and massaging him with 'diaphoretic unctions', followed by two baths and an unnourishing supper.

The greatest of the Arabic doctors, Avicenna (AD 979–1037), promoted plenty of bathing, hard exercise, laxatives and food which is bulky but feebly nutritious, and his work *The Canon of Medicine* lasted 600 years. It was not until the seventeenth century that the first publications dealing solely with weight loss began to appear, and still they were mostly for men and also confined to the very large. After all a certain amount of fatness was regarded as healthy and showing a cheerful temper.

Remember that wonderful book I quoted in the Introduction entitled *The Art of Beauty* by 'A Toilet Specialist', published almost a hundred years ago? She suggests that, as all liquids, even water, are fattening, a salient rule for obesity must be to drink as little as possible (advice that is still going the rounds in misinformed diet books today). She also suggests that the patient's bed should be hard, that lolling about on sofas and easy chairs during the day should be avoided, and that when the weather is too unfavourable for exercise then dumbbells or 'light Indian clubs' should be worked before corsets are put on.

A hundred years before liposuction, doctors already had ideas of how to magic away the flesh. The medical publication *The Lancet* stated on 29 July 1898:

> 'Admiral' Soap is suggested as an external cure for corpulence and obesity. The idea is distinctly novel, and is based apparently upon the solvent action upon fat of the active constituents of animal gall. The *rationale* of the treatment, therefore, is that when the soap is applied locally it is absorbed by the pores of the skin with the result . . . of dispersing the adipose tissue . . . It is a light green soap with pleasant aromatic smell.

One satisfied lady wrote: 'For reducing my bust and hips, also waist measurement, I have found it splendid. Both the two former were enormous, but now are as shapely as I could wish.'

The Toilet Specialist suggests that astringent lotions can be efficacious in drying up and absorbing superfluous adipose tissue, but warns that they leave a laxness of skin, a wrinkled and flabby appearance.

Throughout the 1920s and 1930s, slimming methods were vigorously researched. To give you a flavour of the diversity of theories, let me describe the case of the comic novelist William Gerhardie who, as a young man at that time, was anxious to lose a few pounds in order to impress the ladies. He first followed the latest medical advice, which told him to consume plenty of butter and cream because 'these foods, being easily digested, are not fattening'. When this method failed he procured an extraordinary wheeled gadget for rolling his stomach flat (on his return from a holiday abroad the customs officer regarded this novel contraption with deep suspicion). Gerhardie finally resorted to some marvellous new pills which seemed to do the trick (the weight fell off) – until his agitated mother wrote to tell him she had read that the active ingredient was tapeworm eggs.

It is always easy to make fun of previous generations but, especially given our extraordinary medical sophistication, it seems to me that these days we are more credulous than ever. In order to keep the plethora of slimming methods within reasonable limits, in this digest I'll illustrate the information by using either those examples that are currently popular, or those which have an interesting story attached, or those so totally outrageous that it would be a crime not to include them. If you don't find your favourite among those listed, try doing a critique of your own. But please, please, don't write to tell me about it. After researching this chapter I swear that if I ever see another book about dieting (my own excepted, naturally) I'll go mad!

Back to Basics

Let's get one thing clear right from the start. Whether there are 30,000 or a billion different published slimming methods, there is, ultimately, only one way to lose weight: you must eat less than your body requires. In other words, take in fewer calories than you expend. In the welter of dieting claim and counter-claim, it is often easy to forget this simple fact. Keep it at the forefront of your mind when evaluating new plans and half the battle is won. Factors like metabolism may *seem* to complicate the issue – why it is that beastly Rebecca Crunch who lives across the road can consume three times what I do and still stay skinny – but the rule still applies. The only difference is that somehow, whether by secret midnight jogging sessions or because our metabolic rates are wildly different, Miss Crunch is burning up more calories than I am. So I repeat: no matter how you go about it, whether it's by eating only paper doilies, spending your afternoons in jiggling aerobics, or praying to the Almighty, unless you consume fewer calories than you expend, you don't stand a chance. Creams, wraps, injections, massages, potions, special foods, patches and teas are all gloss. Either they don't work at all, or they work only indirectly by encouraging you to stick to that basic, simple golden rule. For the third time then, in big, bold, capital, centred letters:

IF YOU WANT TO GET RID OF FAT, CALORIES IN MUST BE FEWER THAN CALORIES OUT.

Got the message?

Many diet plan writers haven't.

Occasionally they are just plain dim-witted. Mostly it's because what matters to the writer is not so much whether the plan really works as that we, the buyers, *think* that it works. If the writer, publisher and publicity agents can convince us of that, then they're laughing. Dress up old hat or misconception in the right fancy packaging, and somebody starts making big money.

And incidentally, this is not sour cynicism on my part. Believe me, if there was ever a faint possibility of losing weight more easily than via the calories-in-energy-out rule I'd be jumping up and down with glee.

Of course there are honest, well-intentioned diets, but how to spot them?

How to See Through the Packaging

The important thing to remember is that, despite all self-applauding prose, the clever marketing, and the 200-plus pages of text, the message of the vast majority of diet books can be summed up in one line. The essence of Rosemary Conley's *The Hip and Thigh Diet*, for example, is 'eat less fat and exercise'. The rest of it is padding, some helpful, such as recipes and fat tables, some misinformed, such as the notion that you can spot-reduce fat from hips and thighs. Any dieting expert will tell you that it is not possible to spot-reduce. This is so well known that it crops up a thousand times in the medical literature: it is one of the fundamentals of nutrition. If we cut calories we lose weight – but preferentially from the abdomen, the face and the shoulderblades (and, alas, very often from the bosom). Indeed, women are built in such a way that the very last place they will lose flesh is from their hips and thighs. Nutritional experts Dr Tom Sanders and Peter Bazalgette carried out a study at King's College, London, and once again proved what everybody in the business knew already:

> We're sorry, Rosemary, there is no magic formula, nor has [your weight loss] anything to do with the nature of the diet. If we consume fewer calories, we lose weight. There is no good scientific evidence to show that low-fat diets lead to particular weight-loss from the hips and thighs.

The fact that the very thrust of Conley's book is founded on a mistake – it is, after all, called *The Hip and Thigh Diet* – and, furthermore, that such a basic mistake should have crept past someone who has spent so long in the dieting industry, should in itself make one cautious of believing diet-book claims. See Sanders' and Bazalgette's book *You Don't Have to Diet* for more about Conley's unfortunate mistakes.

Judith Wills' diet books and the *BBC Diet* are also all 'eat less fat and exercise': after all, fats are very high in calories and cutting back on them is one way to satisfy the golden rule.

However, packaging *is* important in helping you to stick to the diet in the first place. Diet promoters devise all sorts of tricks and gimmicks to keep you at it: fixed menus so that you don't have to think what to eat; fixed proportions in an attempt to prevent you eating too much; charts to fill in to record your progress and your goals; an initial very-low-calorie phase to promote rapid weight loss; occasional 'treats'; dull foods to make eating dull; monotonous meal patterns; eating rituals; monitoring by another person; group pressure. Diet-book writers are forever introducing complicating factors to try to make their proposal a little different. Some have come up with the most peculiar ideas. Others have displayed an almost contemptuous lack of inventiveness. Leah Leneman, in *Slim the Vegetarian Way*, proudly boasts of her 'discovery that two teaspoons of vegetable oil is quite sufficient for sautéeing vegetables'. My own contribution is the brilliant discovery that if you eat all your food with chopsticks it makes it last twice as long.

Let's look more closely at some of the more commonly used packaging tricks.

It's Revolutionary! This is a word that should set your alarm bells ringing. Hold on tight to your wallet. The diet *may* be interesting, it might even be helpful, but it is, almost certainly, not 'revolutionary'. Why not? For the simple reason that there's only one way to lose weight. Eat fewer calories than you use up. The only 'revolutionary' element that has been added to this basic physical rule is our understanding of nutrition, which allows us to distinguish an unhealthy from a balanced diet.

This doesn't stop them however. Picking out a random sample of my huge pile I see 'revolutionary' blazoned across half a dozen titles. The very preponderance of the word should make you wary.

There are two types of 'revolutionary' claim. First, those who say they've discovered something brand new which nobody before knew about. It might be a startling scientific fact, an imaginative new method of keeping you on the plan, or just a different page layout. But look closer and you will almost always find that the new fact is just an old fact in new clothes, or a totally wrong 'fact'. *The Hip and Thigh Diet* is, as I have said, eat less fat and exercise, a dietary regimen that has been used from at least the time of Galen onwards.

The Rotation Diet proposes an astounding new way to outwit your metabolism; slimming patches contain a seaweed preparation which is supposed to be absorbed into your blood and speed up metabolism; amino acid pills like Slim-Nite make you 'Shape up while you sleep!'

The other type of 'revolutionary' claim is the reverse of the above. The revolution involves adopting a very old technique. Leslie Kenton shot to fame with her 'revolutionary' *Raw Energy* book, which promoted the eating of all things raw. In my zeal for health and energy I bought it, filled up my cupboards with every possible dried pea and bean that I could lay my hands on which might possibly sprout, crunched through a million carrots and a billion sunflower seeds, and for a week patiently ignored the fact that this was the most inconvenient and unrewarding diet I'd ever been on in my life, before giving up and silently dumping a car bootful of sprouted whatnots in a nearby skip. (They had proliferated at a quite alarming rate: every time I ate one, two more appeared. I still have sprout nightmares.) The trouble with books like this is that although the authors are obviously sincere, what worked well for them does not necessarily work for other people.

Kenton's new book *Biogenics* is 'revolutionary' because she insists we drop everything and start living like a peculiar, predominantly men-only sect that flourished in Palestine between 2 BC and AD 1. It is in the same mould as the previous book: heftily researched, relentlessly enthusiastic, and the idea is that if only we'd eat like these turn-of-the-millennium Palestinians all our troubles would vanish. Kenton is not one to let even-handedness hamper her style. She compares being even 10 lbs overweight to 'lumbering . . . like a self-conscious rhinoceros'. And if any reader should have the temerity to open her mouth in disagreement at this absurdity, Kenton rushes on to declare that 'no matter how much you console yourself with the idea that you are generally healthy, that you do eat well . . . we are not as alive as we could be, nor as beautiful, nor as joyous – and we know it.' So there!

What drivel! Perhaps being 10 lbs overweight if you are 3 ft nothing will turn you into a rhinoceros. I have been 20 lbs over and run and jumped merrily, and could have challenged her to a karate match, a yoga sitting or a session of the splits.

It's Fast! They say the modern obsession with 'instant' everything has to do with nuclear weapons, and a worry that we must grab all we can now, as tomorrow may be too late. Certainly, saying your diet works fast is one of the best ways to get it selling fast. Judith Wills and Miriam Stoppard are among the worst offenders, and both ought to know better. Wills was for ten years editor of *Slimmer* magazine, a publication that repeatedly and correctly points out that high-speed dieting is unhealthy, useless, gets rid only of water and muscle, and that if you want to shed fat, you shouldn't buy any book that promises to lose you more than 2 lbs a week. But curiously, this message does not seem to have got through to Ms Wills, author of such gems as *High Speed Slimming* and *A Flat Stomach in Fifteen Days*. It's amazing how working in the slimming industry seems to give people amnesia.

As a medical doctor, Miriam Stoppard, too, knows full well that *Lose 7 lbs in 7 Days* is nonsense, because 7 lbs off in seven days equals 7 lbs on again before you've had time to try out the new swimsuit. Her idea is that instead of trying to beat the mood-elevating effect carbohydrates have on some people, you should indulge it with 'a potato in its jacket, or a cupful of rice or a plate of dahl'. Because carbohydrates tend to be bulky, it is by eating more of them than anything else that you make yourself feel full without consuming too many calories, though as anyone knows who's tried this sort of approach the feeling is short-lived. This is part of the reason why she also insists that you eat small meals six times a day. Not bad advice, but I swear if I read another diet plan that says 'are you kidding, you actually want me to eat *more* on this diet?' (or words to that effect) I shall scream. No matter what she says, you're going to feel as hungry as hell. And judging by the cover of her book and the predatory look she's giving that apple, I'd say she's pretty hungry too.

According to surveys, most women get their slimming diet plans, especially the high-speed ones, from magazines. Marina Andrews' *Encyclopedia of Slimming Diets* is not, alas, an encyclopedia of popular diets, but a collection of 176 diets that she has published in magazines during her long career as 'an internationally recognized Health, Diet and Beauty Consultant'. They give a good indication of the amusing, quirky and often downright silly diets that magazines are constantly making up, especially around Christmas and in the run-up to summer. They range from one day to two months in duration. Some of them are delightful. I made a beeline for the 'Grapefruit and Champagne Diet', designed to make you feel 'marvellously uplifted'. Alas, you're only allowed one bottle of champagne a day, in six miserly doses, which, she soberly reassures all her more delicate readers, offers very little chance of getting you 'tiddly'. The 'One-Day Inner Cleanliness Diet' permits you eight small glasses of a sort of cheesy Bloody Mary concoction, without the vodka. The 'Prune Diet' has you taking seventy-eight prunes in three days and six glasses of prune juice. If you want to spend three days sitting on the loo, then this is the diet for you! Of her diets, 149 are for one week or less, otherwise known by doctors as dehydration diets.

All the same, if you really want fast weight loss, let me tell you the secret of the permanent weight loss 7 lbs in seven hours diet: go to a Turkish Bath for the afternoon. Then eat dried oats for the rest of your life.

It's Got Scientific Mumbo-Jumbo. The Americans excel at this. We British just don't have the gall to come up with the sort of outrages to nutritional understanding that some of our cousins across the Atlantic go in for. For example, Harvey and Marilyn Diamond, the authors of *Fit For Life* (also 'revolutionary'), have a squeamish obsession with the idea that food gets stuck and rots in the intestine creating toxins that get into the blood and cause disease. This is nonsense, but popular nonsense all the same. De-tox diets thrive on making your perfectly ordinary, healthy digestive processes sound like a nauseating quagmire. In the introduction to this book it is announced that the Diamonds 'have chosen to devote their life to the study of the human body in a way other than the two-dimensional technological approach prevalent in many universities'. In non-PR speak, this means that these two characters are pushing an Eastern kind of pseudoscience, dubbed Siddha Yoga, which they boned up on at the American College of Health Sciences, an unaccredited and correspondence institution in Texas. 'As noted by the National Council Against Health Fraud, the book's only socially redeeming feature is that it may be a good gauge of the nation's ignorance on health and nutrition,' writes Dr Magadau in *The American Journal of Gastroenterology*.

The packaging of Neal Barnard's *Foods that Cause You to Lose Weight: The Negative Calorie Effect* is as crucial in making you part with your money as is the ludicrous claim. It actually comes in a cellophane package, so that you have to spend £8.95 in order to see if this unbelievably wonderful promise is, in fact, believable. Of course it isn't. You knew all along it wasn't, didn't you? If foods existed that actually 'cause you to lose weight' it would have been splashed all over the newspapers long before Barnard had time to reach for his word processor. But Barnard knows the dieter's psychology, and people go on buying such books *just in case*. In fact, as you would expect, his title is a misuse of language. He points out that it takes the body more energy to digest complex carbohydrates than fats, and rushes on to conclude that, therefore, on balance, on a high-carbohydrate diet the body uses up more energy, thus putting an end to podge. But this doesn't mean carbohydrate foods *cause* you to lose weight: eating twice as many isn't going to make you twice as thin. The only thing that causes weight loss is calorie restriction (yawn!). If you restrict calories while eating only pure ghee, you'll do just as well as far as slimming is concerned.

What Barnard means is that you can, calorie for calorie, eat a little more carbohydrate than fat. But how great an effect does this have? Barnard doesn't say. The reason is simple. The effect would be minuscule. In *The Stillman Diet* (also known as the water diet because it requires you to drink eight glasses of fluid a day), the American Dr Stillman used the same argument to favour protein. Since, as for complex carbohydrates, protein molecules are larger than fat molecules, he said up to 30 per cent more energy is used in their digestion than in the case of other foods. Proper scientific studies found that, if anything, it is more like 2 per cent. Let's do a quick calculation to test Stillman's and Barnard's ideas. Digestion accounts for between 5 and 10 per cent of the energy we consume. So, if we compare a 1500-calorie protein-only diet with a similar fat-only diet, the difference in the amount of our daily basic energy requirements used in digestion is 0.2 per cent, which is 3 calories or a little under 1/1000th of a pound of fat.

Gosh.

Just to be on the safe side Stillman has also published the *Quick Inches Off Diet*, a 'spot-reducing' diet very high in carbohydrates, and *forbidding* meat, seafood, poultry, cheeses and eggs.

Judy Manzel's very popular *Beverly Hills Diet* may be one of the most widely condemned diet books in history. This contribution to nutritional misunderstanding was first published in 1980, and invariably gets a lousy mention in any academic article on popular diet books, and sells superbly well. A very high (90 per cent) carbohydrate diet consisting of days and days on fruit only (e.g. only papaya on Monday, only watermelon *plus seeds* on Tuesday, etc.), followed by enormous binges, which you atone for on the morrow by eating just, say, pineapple. And so it goes on: diarrhoea, diarrhoea, SCOFF, diarrhoea, diarrhoea, SCOFF ... 'Manzel, like a sham-fed animal equipped with a gastric fistula allowing food to be shunted out of the body before it reaches the intestines, eats continuously,' stated *The International Journal of Eating Disorders* in an editorial entitled 'The Beverly Hills Eating Disorder: The Mass Marketing of Anorexia Nervosa'.

Manzel is one of the many slimming gurus who is obviously really messed up about food. She started dieting at eight years old, and went downhill from then on. She so upset herself with diet drugs that in ten days without them she once gained 22 lbs. You'd imagine that by the time she got round to writing this book she'd have known a bit about the subject, but the calorific haywire of her life has completely addled her thoughts: body fat is something that has been ingested but not digested, according to her. She confuses feeling empty and being dehydrated, with losing fat. She thinks 'carbs' (carbohydrates) get stuck in your stomach.

Manzel's cycle of bingeing and purging is designed to outwit the body's physiological defences against the effects of dieting. This is the same approach adopted by Martin Katahn's *The Rotation Diet*, which insists that you rotate the amount of calories eaten with the aim of preventing the drop in metabolism that accompanies any significant and prolonged period of calorie restriction: 600 calories for the first three days, 900 for the next four, 1200 for the remaining seven. Repeat this two-week cycle *ad nauseam*. It won't do you the blindest bit of good (if anything, you'd think any self-respecting body would assume you're going loopy, and start piling up reserves in case you get any worse), but it gives you something to concentrate on if you're feeling bored. 'No scientific data shows that this diet works or even how it could work,' remark the ever-patient authors of *Food, Nutrition and Diet Therapy*.

Herman Taller, in *Calories Don't Count*, a famous, mail-order high-fat diet from the Sixties, claims that if the dieter eats the right amount of polyunsaturated fat, taking safflower oil and margarine, this will stimulate the pituitary gland and burn off body fat more effectively. In truth, it does nothing of the sort. All the oil does is to add calories – 124 of them per spoonful. Dr Taller was eventually charged with mail fraud.

It Has Worked for Millions of Other Readers! Testimonials from happy readers have always been popular. They're easy enough to get: most diets work in the short term providing you stick to them.

Nowadays we're all concerned not just that the weight comes off, but that it stays off. That is where statistics come in handy, with diet-book writers throwing in a host of grand sentences and a few figures to show that, contrary to the well-established scientific evidence that diets have a 90 to 95 per cent failure rate, their diet has the most amazing success rate (around 80 per cent seems to be the current fashionable figure). There are two ways to judge this: either the writer is lying, or the writer has a poor grasp of the basic principles of objective statistical research. To claim that a diet has worked for someone, you have to show that after starting the diet the person stayed on it, lost weight, and, having completed it, did not regain the weight. There are all sorts of ways to fudge your results.

Let's say I publish the 'Fountain Pen Diet'. On this plan you drink only bottles of Parker Quink until you either lose the weight you want or end up in hospital. I sell several thousand copies of the diet. Of those, ten readers sit down to write to me. Eight of them love it, the remaining two think it's the most miserable piece of rubbish they've ever had the misfortune to get involved in. But this doesn't mean that the plan has an 80 per cent success rate. All it means is that people have rather generous natures: any author (with the possible exception of Salman Rushdie) will tell you that readers are much more likely to write to you if they like your book than if they don't. In this case, it probably also means that at least eight of my readers were unbalanced. Besides, what do a few letters tell me, anyway? If I knew what the thousands of people who'd begun the diet and didn't write to me thought about it, then I might have a decent amount of evidence, but I'd also soon find that my success rate had plummeted, alas.

As Josie put it:

> I bought this diet book X. It didn't work for me and I know
> at least eight other women who also bought it and are just

the same size. Yet new editions come out saying 80 per cent success rate. I do wonder where all these successful slimmers are. Not one of my many failed friends have been asked for their opinions.

Always bear in mind the old adage 'There are lies, damned lies and statistics'. You can make a statistic out of anything.

Most writers, however, don't bother to justify their claims. They just leap on the 80 per cent bandwagon, and hope you'll believe them. Rosemary Conley is an exception. In the latest edition of *The Complete Hip and Thigh Diet* she declares that she was 'determined to establish the diet's long-term results. My only way of establishing these facts was to write to those dieters whose weight details appeared in my earlier book and who had completed the original questionnaire.' She then gives a page of results showing that her diet has, over a five-year period, lo and behold, a success rate of, yes, wait for it . . . about 80 per cent (76 per cent, to be exact).

On the basis of the very limited information she supplies about the way the research was conducted it is completely impossible to judge the value of the statistic. Her method of soliciting follow-up letters from slimmers who previously got themselves into her earlier bestseller by expressing satisfaction with the diet will not provide an unbiased sample. One possibility is that Conley confined her research to those women who have *remained* on the diet for the duration of five years, and does not include those who began the diet and then stopped. This is an approach used by the manufacturers of Slimfast. Their evidence for long-term weight loss involves people on 'maintenance plans' who return to the full plan if they start to regain weight. Naturally, this is in complete contradiction to what it means to follow a diet plan successfully: a successful diet is one that gets off the fat and, by encouraging you to change your eating habits, keeps it off once the diet is over. Of course, if you look just at those people who are prepared to spend the rest of their lives on the diet, eating only a piddlesome amount, you're going to find that most of them remain skinny. But in this case they are still on the diet, and, since the diet is not over, it can't yet be said to have succeeded or failed. However, the vast majority of people don't have the body and metabolism that enable them to do this. The vast majority finish the diet and go back to eating exactly as they did before beginning. This is why the statistics are so bad, and why the only slimming approach that works does not concentrate on greatly reducing calories for quick weight loss, but on changing eating habits gradually. However, if Conley has made this mistake, then what's surprising is not that her result is as high, but that it's as low at 76 per cent.

The Carbohydrate Addict, by Drs Rachel and Richard Heller, has, we are told, a greater than 80 per cent long-term success rate, but says nothing about how this statistic was arrived at. *The Cambridge Diet,* now infamous for its high failure rate, (i.e. very few people lose weight for the long term) was, we were confidently informed by its inventor and publicist, Dr Alan Howard, at least 60 per cent successful.

Oh, and just because a celebrity recommends a product or plan doesn't necessarily mean anything more than that they've been paid a good whack. Remember Jerry Hall, paid to promote Bovril, who had her contract cancelled after she uttered the immortal lines, 'You think ah *eat* that stuff? Ah black mah boots with it', or words to that effect. Most ungenerous about such a venerable British foodstuff.

Doctors Love It! I referred above to Dr Alan Howard, a highly respected doctor in Cambridge whose papers on dieting frequently appeared in major international academic journals. And yet his commercial product *The Cambridge Diet* has been widely condemned. At best it should be treated with great caution. In an article on fad diets in *Postgraduate Medicine* Professor Friedman, of the University of Wisconsin Medical School, writes that 'most people undertake the program without medical supervision. This is extremely dangerous. The Food and Drug Administration and the American Society of Bariatric Physicians warn that such very-low-calorie diets pose a significant health hazard if they are not supervised by a physician.' Moral: Just because the author is a 'Dr', don't think that means he or she must have the right answer. Also, make sure you check what sort of 'Dr' the author is. This is easiest on American books where a medical doctor has MD after his or her name, standing for 'Medical Doctor'. If the author is, instead, Dr So-and-so PhD, that means he or she is *not* a medical doctor. A 'doctorate' is an academic qualification, but it can be in any subject – it might be in gold-mining, for all you know.

A recent so-called breakthrough in America which will probably soon wend its way over here (at least in terms of commercial strategy, if not in detail) is a diet plan produced by the grandly titled United Sciences of America, Incorporated. It has received a lot of attention because of its slick, hugely expensive marketing campaign and its endorsement by a scientific advisory board composed of internationally renowned doctors and scientists. The plan is supposed to provide 'optimal nutrition' for Americans. And yet, curiously, this supposedly 'optimal' formulation includes 300 times the recommended daily amount of thiamine, 250 times the recommended daily amount of ascorbic acid and 133 times the recommended daily amount of vitamin E, and is completely lacking in two essential minerals, phosphorus and iron. Oh, and it was quickly discovered that the members of the scientific board had been awarded substantial 'grants' by the company for their favours. Writes one nutritionist, 'this diet is but the latest example of "yuppie" pseudoscience . . . [and the] secret-formula "fiber energy bar" in keeping with the great tradition of the American medicine-man huckster.'

How the Packaging Comes Together

Before concluding this section, I want to take a closer look at one of the most popular diet books, to show just how misleading the packaging can be. I have chosen Judith Wills' *Size 12 in 21 Days* (published in 1993) as a good example.

My first thought when I picked it up was size 12 *from what?* Size 12 from size 18, 22, 24? In twenty-one days? My second thought concerned the skinny woman on the front. A cursory flick through revealed scores of photos of Ms Wills, looking not only skeletally thin but, to me, distinctly unhealthy. A second model demonstrating exercises showed a ribcage that would not have looked out of place in a prison camp. Evidently this was going to be one of those desperate remedies for anybody who wants to outdo Twiggy *and* Kate Moss.

I read the introduction. I had to read it twice. Surely it must be a joke? The book purports to be 'a celebration of the curvier woman'. I read on:

> There's no doubt about it, thin is no longer in. For the woman of the '90s, her shape to be is . . . well . . . shapely.
> And so *Size 12 in 21 Days* is the first diet book for women

who don't want to be thin. It's written for women like you and me – women who want to look good but aren't afraid to be female. We want a bust, a waist, hips and a bottom. We want the shape that fits into – and looks great in – a size-12 dress . . . those stretchy leggings need a bottom, the low-cut tops need a bust, and all those lycra dresses need curves, not bones.

This is the book of an unusually skinny woman kidding herself that she is 'rounded', or at least trying to kid us.

The diet itself promises 'two dress sizes in just three weeks'. 'Size 12 is within the grasp of every out-of-shape woman, whether you're a 14, 16 or more.' (Well, yes, let's also say that £100,000 is well within the grasp of every out-of-pocket woman whether she's got a hundred pounds, a thousand pounds or ten thousand pounds in the bank.) It is only when you get to page ten that she concedes that

> if you're very tall, say, 5′ 8″ (1.73m) or over, it will work to reduce you from a 16 or an 18 down to a 14, which may well be your perfect size.

Ah, and here's the sophistry. If you're very large, you simply have to 'repeat the programme'. In other words, size 12 in twenty-one days is not what she means, she means losing one or two dress sizes in twenty-one days:

> If you came to the programme needing to lose more than one or two dress sizes, you can if you wish repeat the whole programme until you are down to your target weight. It is perfectly safe for the long term.

In short, you can get yourself down to a size 12 if you keep going on this crash diet until you are a size 12, and you may, if you feel so inclined, not that it's of any significance, calculate the time it takes you to do so in terms of three-week multiples. And another thing: it turns out in the 'how I discovered this revolutionary diet' section that Wills was already well within her limit on the height–weight charts when she dreamed it up. All that bothered her was that after the birth of one of her children she had an unduly large waist (indeed, looking at the photos, her waist appears still to be the only non-skinny part of her). So she's not talking about general loss of weight, but simply about reducing a postpartum stomach by crash dieting.

I was getting angrier and angrier as I read: she panders to and provokes desperation. Her plan, she promises, will result in:

> more vitality and energy . . . whiter eyes, healthier gums and better, clearer skin. Longer term, hair may become glossier, nails grow stronger, and so on.
>
> Many minor, and not so minor, ailments will improve or clear up altogether because of a combination of better diet and exercise. PMT, fluid retention, low blood sugar, digestive problems, constipation and other niggling problems can be helped through a good, healthy diet.

Even for standard diet stuff this is on the full side. Healthy eating will do what she claims of it, but her diet will not promote healthy eating. She then goes on: 'On the 21 day diet you will learn good eating habits and overcome problems such as bingeing.' In my case, I stuck it for 4 days by which time I was so hungry, I rushed out and bought a mountain of food and gobbled it.

Let's see what's actually being offered.

We have a 'tough start' of 600 calories a day. Okay, it's only for two days, I won't complain.

> You will find, after two days of eating lovely, fresh, low-salt, low-fat foods, that you have literally given your taste buds a crash course in enjoying good, healthy foods rather than fatty, salty, oversweet foods.

This is inane. You cannot educate yourself to 'healthy eating' in two days – not even in two weeks, and not necessarily in two months. The only thing you'll manage to do is increase your cravings for all the 'forbiddens'.

After this 600-calorie blitz we are assured 'the rest of the first week will be a doddle for you calorie-wise because you will now be allowed 1100 calories a day'. No, Ms Wills, it won't be a doddle and, what's more, weight loss of 6 lbs in a week will be mostly fluid and muscle tissue, with proportionately little fat – as Ms Wills should know only too well, because for ten years she was editor of

Slimmer magazine. Those dieters who fail will blame themselves and end up with lower self-esteem than when they started.

Week two. Reduce the calories again! Is this woman joking? Down to 950 a day now. No prizes for guessing what week three involves. Down again to 800 calories. But, 'I promise you that you won't feel hungry'. I wish one could go to court on promises.

The really interesting twist to all this is that just a few years previously, in 1989, Wills published *The Junk Food Diet* (I bought it in my bookshop last year.) In this book she has written a swingeing condemnation of – guess what? High speed dieting.

Over the space of seven paragraphs she damns crash dieting utterly. The only successful way to slim is to do it slowly, she exclaims. Crash dieting is a waste of time, it is very hard to keep up for more than a week, after which most dieters give up and feel a failure, and within two days of ending such a plan you will put on 3 lbs. Oh, and she also points out that you might be threatening your life because you are losing tissue from vital organs such as your heart, instead of losing fat.

In correspondence with Ms Wills, she says that her views have changed since she wrote that book, although she still believes that living on less than an average of around 1,000 calories a day over a period of time is both ineffective and probably very dangerous. But what is *Size 12 in 21 Days* if not a high-speed slimming plan which insists you live on less than an average of around 1,000 calories a day over an extended period – i.e. a crash diet, by her own definition? 600 calories for two days, 1100 for five days, and 950 and 800 calories, respectively, for a week each. A simple twiddle with my calculator shows that to be an average of 902.381 calories per day. My stomach grumbles at the very thought of it. This is the diet programme which, if you wish, you may 'repeat ... until you are down to your target weight' since it is 'perfectly safe for the long term'.

Oh dear, oh dear, Ms Wills.

I think you've got the idea by now. Slimming books are exercises in *advertising*; as such, they are often clever and amusing. As far as losing weight goes you should be **very, very careful** about what you believe.

So, having looked at the packaging, let me now look at the diets themselves in more detail.

THE DIETS

Fasting Diets: 0 Calories

The simplest type of diet is, unsurprisingly, to eat nothing at all. In fasting, which became a bit of a fad at the beginning of the century, all you have is water, though some approaches allow fruit juices. In this manner you can lose up to a pound a day, and the remarkable thing is that after about three days your feelings of hunger diminish, which is why these diets acquired popularity. In the Thirties they went out of fashion, but were resurrected again in 1959. All seemed to be going along swimmingly when the people on fasting diets started dying suddenly. Oops! Starved of input, the body had, in effect, eaten itself alive until there was not enough tissue left in the heart and other vital organs to keep them going any longer. This reminds me of that nice little story about a man who was training his donkey to eat less and less so that by degrees it would require no food at all. He had very nearly accomplished his aim when, to his bitter disappointment, the donkey died.

For short periods, fasting has no serious physical side effects, provided you're healthy to begin with and provided you keep up your liquid intake; but then neither is it beneficial for weight loss, since it will all come back the moment you start eating and drinking again. The American hunger artist Henry Tanner lost 36 lbs on a total fast lasting forty days (some suspected him of cheating), and regained over half of it back in three days of normal eating. Nevertheless, millions of people regularly starve themselves as part of religious fasts, and claim even to derive spiritual benefit from the process. Some historians believe that the frequency with which nuns in the middle ages saw visions had more to do with prolonged fasting than with their spirituality.

I have several friends who obviously do feel a lot better after a short fast, although they say you must be prepared to endure a day or two of headaches and spottiness ('the toxins coming out', or some such). But remember: longer-term fasts are distinctly dodgy. *Never undertake one by yourself. Always consult a doctor.*

Very-Low-Calorie Diets (VLCDs): 200–800 Calories

VLCDs were invented with the hope of providing similar rapid weight loss to that of fasting diets without killing off the patient in the process. They usually come as a powdered drink which you substitute for normal meals for the duration of the plan.

Their history has been a bit of a hit-and-miss affair.

The difficulty is supplying sufficient nutrients for good health, with the minimum calories. No one really knows what the body needs to live on, not least because bodily requirements vary greatly from person to person. The only way to find out is to make a guess and see: if the patient dies, you've left something out.

The aptly named *Last Chance Diet* was one of the early misses. Released in 1976, the principal ingredients of the 500-calorie-a-day powder were predigested collagen and animal-hide gelatin. It seemed a remarkable success until the following year when people started dying again. Drat! 58 people lost their lives due to this inadequate concoction. The silly old inventors hadn't put in enough essential amino acids, and the rapacious human body had once more eaten itself alive.

Undaunted, nutritionists at Cambridge University came up with the *Cambridge Diet*, which had 170 fewer calories (that's right, only 330 calories!) and a lot of very impressive scientific research to back it up and prove it was a good thing. The inventor of this one promised an average weight loss of around $4\frac{1}{2}$ lbs a week, which is about $2\frac{1}{2}$ lbs more than health and success demands. The American government promptly condemned it as a 'serious risk to health' and tried to get it banned. Originally used only in hospital for people considered dangerously obese, then by mail order, these days you can get it through a local 'counsellor' who will visit you at home. One friend of mine on the *Cambridge Diet* lasted two months, only to find, when she attempted to start eating again, that her body simply would not accept food. For several weeks she was violently ill. Other women have been known to become addicted to these diets, and have had to wean themselves off them as they would drugs. The human body is not designed to cope with such massive, swift weight loss.

Oprah Winfrey announced on her TV show in November 1988 that she'd lost 67 lbs using Optifast. The world gawped, clapped and stood aghast, and the switchboard at Sandoz Nutrition (the manufacturers of the 400-calorie-a-day powder) went crazy. They received over a million phone calls following that brilliant piece of free publicity. Then Oprah's weight returned. Exactly two years later, on her show entitled 'The Pain of Regain', a re-enlarged Winfrey declared that 'if you lose weight on a diet . . . sooner or later you'll gain it back'. Indeed, research has shown that VLCDs have a success rate as low as 0.25 per cent. Nevertheless, like the rest of us, Winfrey finds it difficult not to keep on trying, steadily mucking her health up more and more. At the time of writing she's thin again. Personally I think she looked her best – and her most distinctive – at her middle weight, neither very fat nor very thin.

VLCDs should not be used by children, adolescents, pregnant women or the elderly, or by people with gout, heart disease, hypertension or diabetes – the very diseases, in fact, which are usually associated with extreme obesity, the only condition for which VLCDs are recommended! Never even think about a VLCD without consulting your doctor.

So, like fasting, VLCD diets have proved a bit of disappointment. The next brilliant idea was meal replacements. On these you drink your VLCD as before, but add a proper meal (just one a day) to the diet as well, and maybe throw in a 'nutrition' bar for fun. Also you can sell these things over the counter (goody, goody!). Boots Shapers and NutraSlim, Limmits, Carnation Slender, Slimfast are all examples. *Which?* compared thirteen of the most popular plans and found all to be unbalanced, misinformed and to cost considerably more than a similar quantity of normal food.

In their thorough and convincing book, *You Don't Have to Diet*, the nutritionists Dr Tom Sanders and Peter Bazalgette investigate these formulations closely and conclude that it would be much better for you (not to mention much more appetizing than that awful powdered gloop) to replace each of your normal meals by a baked potato and cottage cheese, or a poached egg and spinach on toast, or a ham and tomato wholemeal roll, and the like. These provide about the same number of calories and are much, much cheaper. I personally have never seen the appeal of liquid meal replacements, since if one's consuming 250 or so calories it seems to me plain daft not to enjoy it as food.

Restricted Diets: 800 Calories Plus

Now we enter the big time. It is in this region that most diet books and articles scrabble around trying to find a niche, though it's generally agreed that a safe diet with some chance of working must include at least 1000 calories per day. Given the golden rule that the only way to lose weight is to eat fewer calories, diet books ought to be simple to categorize: either mild, medium or severely restricted, or useless. But diet-book writers are as canny as a troop of monkeys, approaching the subject from every imaginable angle, so that even professional nutritionists sometimes find it hard to make sense of the matter. After much thought, and on the assumption that most of my readers are lay people rather than nutritionists, I have decided on four basic divisions according to commercial type: Special Ingredient Diets, Balanced Diets, Unbalanced Diets, and Psychological and Spiritual Diets. A fifth type – Very Peculiar Diets, such as *Fit for Life* and *The Beverly Hills Diet* – I will not discuss separately, in part because they have no unifying characteristic beyond peculiarity, but largely because they are so entertaining that I've used the most prominent examples to illustrate other parts of this digest.

Type One: Special Ingredient Diets

Let's make it clear right at the beginning: there are some foods that are better for you than others; there are some foods that will impair digestion in the gut, or give you diarrhoea, or make you sick, and so limit the number of calories you manage to absorb; and there are some foods that sound just so convincingly fat-bashing that they distract you from realizing that the real reason you're losing weight on so-and-so's special ingredient diet is because you're eating less. *But there are no foods that cause weight loss.*

Not that this has ever bothered the diet-mongers. When it comes to inventing fabulous slimming foods, the human imagination leaves no ingredient unturned. It might be something exotic, as in *The Lecithin, B6, Apple Cider Vinegar, and Kelp Diet* (ingredients as stated), which gains its appeal by blinding you with science – after all, these ingredients are odd enough for most of us to be prepared to believe that they will cause magic weight loss. Believe me instead: they don't.

It might be something ordinary, as in the numerous spin-offs of the 'Grapefruit Diet', such as the *Mayo Clinic Diet*, which threw in tomato juice and eggs for good measure; or something downright peculiar as in the *21st Century Diet* (quails' eggs and peppers). A remarkable case discussed before the Royal Society in 1757 concerned a man who had lost 28 lbs during a two-year period by eating a quarter of 1 oz of mild castile soap daily: that's roughly a bar of soap a month to lose a little over 1 lb in weight. Did he eat it raw? Grated? Sprinkled with lemon juice? In a stew? No wonder he needed to reduce – he was capable of eating anything. However, it is never good to be judgemental without doing a little bit of private research, so I duly cooked up a chicken and soap curry and invited a very unpleasant man from work around to supper, myself pleading vegetarianism. I have to admit, he ate everything on his plate without a murmur. But I never did discover if he lost weight.

The Rice Diet was invented in the 1940s to lower blood pressure, but it has reappeared as a weight-loss diet: you eat rice and fruit until it becomes too awful to go on. The supposed (and completely fictitious) weight-loss properties of grapefruit were first shouted from the rooftops in the 1920s and reappeared again in the 1970s. These days pineapples have also been, equally unjustly, applauded. Caffeine, by making you jittery, uses up a few extra calories indirectly and so, lo and behold, many diet pills and potions use caffeine extract as their principal ingredient.

Honey is a special ingredient. The irrepressible Barbara Cartland has written a book more or less on the subject called *The Magic of Honey* ('Including New Wonder Diet', says my revised edition). On the cover there's a terrifying photo of Miss C. bedecked with jewels and defying you to deny honey's myriad virtues. Cartland's delicate, beautiful married friend Serena complains coyly that men 'are often very exhausted in the evenings'. 'Honey is the answer!' exclaims Cartland, who is not in the least bit delicate about such matters. If 'genital function' is really bad, these rotters are encouraged to eat a special concoction of multivitamins, GEV-E-TABS, mysterious stuffs called Celaton CH₃ Tri-Plus (the reason why 'last year I wrote twenty-four books'), Keitafo Banlon ('communicated secretly from the Chinese Imperial Palace') and Ginseng – two, one, four and two tablets, respectively. Honey is also critical for health, healing, beauty, nerves, and general all-over happiness, which I am quite prepared to believe if for no better reason than that I love bees. After 114 pages of break-neck honey-praising, Barbara Cartland finally reveals her 'New Wonder Diet'. The most remarkable thing about it is that it has nothing to do with honey at all. It is just an ordinary low-carbo-hydrate diet, with a particular emphasis on banning sugars. But honey is almost pure carbohydrate in sugar form. So, curiously, it's an *anti*-honey diet! However, meat is a special slimming food, Cartland assures us. After all, 'Have you ever seen a fat tiger?' Indeed, next to honey, meat is Cartland's favourite food: she finds vegetarians nervy, anaemic and limp in more ways than one.

High-fibre diets have a tendency to be special-ingredient diets. Dietary fibre (also called bulk or roughage) is the part of leaves, seeds, roots, fruits and plants not digested. It is good for you because it helps to carry food and waste efficiently through your body. Too little fibre and you get constipation and a variety of nasty ailments associated with the digestive system. But fibre is not a miracle slimming food. It may slightly limit the number of calories you digest by binding together other food so that it is absorbed by the body more slowly. On a very-high-fibre diet, the effect of this malabsorption on weight loss is estimated to be, at most, of the order of an ounce a week. Eating bran flakes like a combine harvester is not going to make you thin.

Audrey Eyton's *F-Plan*, the original popular high-fibre diet book, came out in 1982, and went on to become the best-selling diet book in the world: 810,000 copies within three weeks of publi-cation (wish I'd thought of it first). The politician David Owen was a self-confessed follower, so was Terry Wogan, and even my builder admitted losing weight on it. Eyton claimed not only that fibre was a slimming food but also that it fills you up with non-calorific matter so that you don't feel hungry. This last claim is true in the short term; but stomachs stretch so that they can take in more food and thus get the energy you require for day-to-day functioning. Moral: never underestimate a stomach.

High-fibre buffs are obsessed with their stools. 'If you're indeli-cate like I am, and peer down the loo,' enthused Eyton, 'you'll see that there's a lot of sweetcorn in your stools – if you eat sweetcorn, that is – along with other foods high in fibre like peas and beans.' A healthy, fibrous, applaudable emission should be voluminous, soft, sticky and jagged at the edges, like those of Africans, who eat fibre by the bucketful, not the miserable little rabbit-droppings most Europeans produce.

In fact, there are not two categories of stools but six. I will repeat them here because I know just how fascinated we all (secretly) are by such matters:

1) Separate hard lumps, like nuts.
2) Sausage-shaped but lumpy.
3) Like a sausage or snake but with cracks on its surface.
4) Like a sausage or snake, smooth and soft.
5) Soft blobs with clear-cut edges.
6) Fluffy pieces with ragged edges, a mushy stool.

This fascinating piece of information appears in Gilly Smith's *Fibrenetics*, a more recent high-fibre book. It is straightforward, very informative, and after a few pages I found myself rushing downstairs for an apple. Sensibly, she does not sell high fibre so much on its dubious slimming credentials as on its very well-established health ones, and on the principle that a healthy, balanced diet provides the best route to weight loss. If that's her on the cover she certainly is extraordinarily thin, but very elegant and unusual with it – more in the intriguing mould of Morticia Adams than the usual ghastly grinning bimbo. She reveals some new information about pre-menstrual tension which is well worth looking at if you're a sufferer. The recipes at the back are all from British restaurants.

Type Two: Balanced Diets

As medical evidence grows against the value of dieting – and against high-speed, unbalanced dieting in particular – so does the number of books advocating a more gradual, less hysterical approach to slimming. These concentrate on a reduction of the number of calories you eat, but do not focus on one particular type of food. Beloved of slimming magazines, in book form such dietary regimens are often just a series of calorie-counted, balanced menus with a long introduction tacked on. In my experience, most of us buy the books but never follow the menus for very long.

Balanced slimming diets offer a far better chance of permanent weight loss than unbalanced ones, since they allow you normal eating patterns and the full range of foods. But don't expect to lose more than a pound or two a week and, if you are to keep the weight off, you must assume that the diet makes a permanent change in your eating habits. If you're exercising as well, you may find that though you lose in girth you may even gain a little in weight, because muscle weighs more than fat. This is both healthy and desirable.

I recommend Debra Waterhouse's *Outsmarting the Female Fat Cell,* which is a sensible, intelligent, relaxed, reassuring plan, though rather complicated to work out. Best of all it's full of pictures of darling little fat cells with 'ON' and 'OFF' written in them, and things like 'fat cell on a diet' and 'sedentary fat cell' inscribed beneath. I like the look of Deborah Waterhouse on the cover, too. She's a proper size, fully clad, and not half-swivelled round, arching herself at the reader in a desperate attempt to show off an insubstantial waist or thigh.

Another good example of a balanced diet book is the *Super Foods Diet Book* by Michael Van Straten and Barbara Griggs. The text is calm, unusually well informed, and the menus included are delicious. Van Straten and Griggs' aim is not to produce skimpy meals, but enjoyable, substantial, healthy ones which will encourage your body to work efficiently without feeling hungry. It's a good sign in itself that they open with an apt quote from Montaigne:

> On those who prescribe diets: if they do no other good, they prepare their patients for death, by gradually undermining and cutting off their enjoyment of life.

Super Foods is loosely based on the Hay system of food combining, invented by the American doctor William Howard Hay in the Thirties. This demands that carbohydrates be eaten separately from proteins, and both separately from fruit if you are to maintain a healthy alkaline/acid balance. The system has become particularly fashionable in the last few years, partly because Fergie, the Duchess of York, uses it. Primarily, however, the object of the Hay method is not to lose weight, but to gain health, and though it is generally thought of in the medical profession as a pile of hooey, there are many people who claim it to be the most wonderful thing that ever happened to them. These two views are not necessarily incompatible. Hay's *theory* is definitely haywire: most foods, particularly plant foods, on which Hay was especially keen, are already a combination of proteins and carbohydrates, so you can't separate them, and the alkali/acid stuff makes the body sound like it was a frail flower of a thing, rather than the resilient and highly efficient mechanism it is. But *in practice* it appears to have some good results with some people, for whatever reason. I was sceptical until I asked the opinion of a marvellous allergy specialist I know: she confirmed that the Hay system has excellent results with some people. My friend Brenda, who lives in Italy, is a devoted fan, and is fit, healthy, energetic and beset by appreciative Roman lovers. This might have more to do with Brenda's oodles of *je ne sais quoi* than with the Hay system, but who knows?

Kathryn Marsden's *The Food Combining Diet* is (at time of writing) the most recent and certainly the most popular Hay book. It's part of a series, which also includes, by different authors, *Food Combining for Health* and *Food Combining for Vegetarians*. Praise the Lord, these books don't have photos of skinny adolescents or calorie-exhausted authors on the front. At one point Marsden remarks, in justification of her programme, that 'our hunter-gatherer ancestors certainly didn't indulge in the kind of mixed food fiasco we are familiar with today', to which Dr Sanders, in *You Don't Have to Diet*, retorts yes, 'but if health is the issue, their average life expectancy was 28; ours is almost three times as much'. Touché!

Two recent diet plans written by highly respected cooks are John Tovey's *Having a Binge on a Diet* and Prue Leith's rather stricter (in terms of calories) *The Sunday Times Slim Plan*. The best thing about Leith's book is she's got colour photos of what each meal option looks like, so you can pick out the biggest at a glance. But the plan is monumentally complicated, and makes use of scores of little symbols so that you can calculate the food values, and so forth. I personally feel this approach is death to any long-term dieting unless you are of a very slavish disposition. What one wants is to understand the rules of healthy eating and then try and forget about food and simply enjoy it as one pleasant aspect of life. Leith includes a helpful discussion of healthy take-away and restaurant options.

With John Tovey I felt an immediate affinity. Here is someone who loves food but has had to lose weight – lots of it. He writes amusingly on 'how he managed to diet away 3 stone without living on a regime of lettuce leaves and mineral water', and suggests lots of ways of eating healthily without in any way conveying that terrible dieting desperation. There are good recipes too. Best of all it's a reasonable book: you believe him.

There are numerous other examples of balanced diet books.

Vegetarian diets are often balanced, the author being far too taken up with weaning you off meat to try to mess up the rest of your food supply as well. Beware those with an excessively sanctimonious tone, and ensure the plan includes plenty of protein from dairy produce and (especially if vegan) beans, nuts, pulses and potatoes.

How to spot other nutritionally balanced slimming plans? They are usually written in calm language, do not advocate severely restricting any particular type of food, and tend to focus less on the ingredients of your food and more on ways of adjusting your eating habits. If you are interested in long-term, healthy weight loss these are the only ones to consider.

Type Three: Unbalanced Diets

Crudely speaking, a healthy diet should get a little around half of its calories from carbohydrates, about a third from fats, and the remainder from proteins. Unbalanced diets therefore focus on reducing or increasing one or two of the categories, at the expense of the other. So the 'inventor' of such a plan has six options: low or high fat; low or high carbohydrate; and low or high protein. In practice, every such diet is categorizable under more than one of these headings since by tampering with one food type, it ends up tampering with the others. In my brief survey, below, I've listed the diets according to the food type on which the most emphasis is placed.

One of the main 'advantages' of this type of dieting is that the body's response to the nutritional imbalance results in rapid initial weight (not fat) loss due to dehydration. On diets where this does not happen, you will often find that there's a three-day semi-fast to start you off. Another advantage, from the marketing point of view, is that they have the convincing ring of jargon about them. You just can't help feeling that a low-fat diet must mean that fats are what make you fat, or that a high-protein diet is successful because proteins somehow 'cause' you to lose weight. Neither is true.

The main disadvantage of unbalanced diets is side effects. They are unbalanced, after all.

Low-Carbohydrate Diets: I grew up on the conventional wisdom that potatoes, pasta and bread are the arch enemies of weight loss, but nutritionists now know that to be completely wrong. The body desperately needs such carbohydrates to keep itself supplied with blood sugar. When deprived, various emergency plans have to be adopted, such as breaking down muscle tissue and producing what are known as ketones from the fat molecules, which result in a 'fruity' breath and a 'woozy' feeling characteristic of this sort of diet. An advantage of low-carbohydrate diets is that the production of ketones, at least at first, makes hunger less intense. A disadvantage is that carbohydrates (which include both sugar and wheat) are basic to many delicious foods and dishes, and that constipation is common (due to lack of fibre, a type of carbohydrate), as are nausea and fatigue. Breaking down your muscle tissue is never a good idea, not least because it leads to a higher fat ratio in your body.

The most famous example of a low-carbohydrate diet is *The Scarsdale Diet*, by Herman Tarnower. One of the more unlucky diet promoters, Dr Scarsdale, though no great beauty, was hacked to death with a hatchet by a jealous lover. He was also fifteen pounds overweight according to his own tables. *Dr Atkin's Diet, The Drinking Man's Diet* and *The Pennington Diet* are other examples of low-carbohydrate diets.

Low-carbohydrate diets went out of fashion during the Eighties, but are making something of a comeback with the idea that some people are overweight because they are carbohydrate 'addicts'. Eating buns and plateful of pasta in creamy sauce gives them a high, followed by a low, followed by another sticky bun and a plateful of spaghetti. An example of this breed is *The Carbohydrate Addict's Diet*, by Rachel and Richard Heller, who gain and lose hundreds of pounds within the space of a few lines, repeat this over the extent of several pages (exhausting stuff to read, I can tell you), before they finally decide to stop gorging on carbohydrates and sit down and write a 'revolutionary' diet book instead. Whether or not the addiction theory is up to much, is, nevertheless, hotly debated. If you do find it difficult to stop eating pasta and puddings, and perhaps feel sleepy after doing so, then this sort of book is probably worth looking at.

High-Carbohydrate Diet: The basic principle of this sort of diet is 'fill 'em up with food that ain't got much in it'. Some are reasonable (in Britain, the average person eats about half the recommended amount of carbohydrates, so even if such diets are nothing special in the weight-loss bag of tricks, they are good for your health), others are not.

Rose Elliot's contribution to the genre is a case in point. I have a well-used copy (sticky blobs on every page) of her *Complete Vegetarian Cookbook*, but I was surprised to find how very disappointing is her vegetarian *The Green Age Diet*. Though I'm all in favour of 'helping to save the planet' I cannot recommend it at all. She expects you to lose a stone (i.e. seven times the medically recommended limit) in the first week, and her goal weights are among the lowest I've come across; they rank as significantly underweight according to even the severest of insurance company charts, take no account of age or frame size and offer only a single weight, instead of a range. At 5 ft 9 ins I'm supposed to weigh 9 st 1 lb, which, judging from what I looked and felt like at 10 st 7 lbs, is appalling. Yes, of course there are healthy women this tall and this thin, but it cannot do for all of us, willy nilly. In several instances her weights are getting into the degree of skinniness which has been found to be associated with a considerable increase in mortality. Elliot herself acknowledges that even she's never yet managed to reach her own goal weight! In fact, the charts are taken uncritically ('slavishly' would be nearer the mark) from the American *Rice Diet*, dismissed as a quack diet by the medical profession in the USA, and based on a plan first proposed by a Dr Walter Kempner fifty years ago.

Although the latest medical thinking is that a healthy diet is rich in complex carbohydrates, you can go too far. Very-high-carbohydrate diets tend to be dubiously low in proteins, salt, iron, essential fatty acids and fat-soluble vitamins. Hunger (which returns quickly after a meal – your body soon realizes it's been duped with feeble food) and boredom are common side effects.

The most amusing high-carbohydrate diet I've come across is the one proposed by Shelly Bovey in *Being Fat Is Not a Sin*. Since it doesn't matter a toot whether you cut calories by eating only grapefruit or extra-thick Devonshire clotted cream, she proposes the fail-safe (provided you stick to it) Delicious Doughnut Diet (approximately 1100 calories):

> *Breakfast* – cup of black coffee or tea, half a grapefruit with sugar substitute, thin piece of wholemeal bread or toast smeared with low-fat spread and Marmite, if liked.
> *Elevenses* – cup of black coffee or tea and a sticky, sugary, jammy, FATTENING doughnut!
> *Lunch* – poached egg on spinach, small slice of melon. No-cal drink (Cola, etc.) or black coffee or tea.

Tea – another doughnut!

Supper – two ounces white fish, large salad with lettuce, chopped raw cabbage, celery, tomato, chives, mint and parsley. Dress with tarragon vinegar.

Later in the evening – hunger pangs? Finish off the day with a cup of black coffee and comfort any first day dieting blues with YET ANOTHER doughnut! And you can eat three more tomorrow.

Low-Fat Diets: Low-fat diets became popular in the Eighties, the most celebrated British version being Rosemary Conley's *Hip and Thigh* series, and in America, *The Pritkin Diet*. Such diets have been used for millennia, but it was the cholesterol and heart disease scare that really got them going recently, and now they abound. *The BBC Diet* and Judith Wills' *High Speed Slimming* are two others in this category. In fact, nowadays most new diets involve reducing fat, although not all make it the focus of their plan. I looked at Wills in the packaging section, above. Let's now take a dekko at Conley.

Rosemary Conley's *Hip and Thigh Diet* is one of the most high-profile diets currently available. There are all sorts of clever little bits of packaging involved here, and I had an interesting time with a medical friend dissecting its claims bit by bit. Writes Conley:

> This revolutionary diet plan, which I had hit upon completely by accident in February 1986 when diagnosed as having a gallstone problem. I was forced on to a low-fat diet, which not only enabled me to avoid major surgery at that time but also had the extraordinary side-effect of reducing my hips and thighs by a great many inches.

But, wait a minute: Conley was working in the slimming business well before her gall bladder operation came up. Indeed, in 1972 she founded the SAGG, Slimming and Good Grooming, organization, later sold it to IPC Magazines Ltd and was appointed Director of Successful Slimming Clubs. Now, the low-fat diet, far from being a diet which had remarkably escaped everybody's imagination until she stumbled on it 1986, was known to even the ancient Greeks. Furthermore, you *cannot* spot-reduce hips and thighs. If anything, fat comes preferentially off the abdomen. And even if you could, it would probably be bad for you, since it would increase your waist-to-hip ratio. You'd think that anyone with her extensive association with the slimming industry would be only too aware of these basic facts. A quick look in the library reveals something else that Rosemary is too modest to mention, namely, that *before* her gall bladder revelation she had written two other much less successful diet books, also emphasizing the need to reduce fats. In *Eat Yourself Slim*, however, she acknowledges that small amounts of fat 'are essential to good health', whereas by the time she published the *Hip and Thigh Diet* her zeal for fashionable androgyny had outweighed her concerns for health, and her list of forbidden fatty foods runs to two pages.

The typical Briton gets about 40 per cent of her calories from fat; in America, about 50 per cent. A healthy diet should have 20–30 per cent. Low-fat diets sometimes go as low as 5 per cent, and in extreme cases may try to eliminate fat altogether, which deprives your body of essential fatty acids and fat-soluble vitamins. Too little vitamin A (found in butter, milk and cheese) can result in increased risk of breast cancer. In countries where diets are very low in fat, night blindness, eye lesions and complete blindness are correspondingly more common. Vitamin D (oily fish is the best source) protects against osteoporosis; too little can result in bone softening in adolescents, pregnant women and the elderly. (However, if you're on a very low fat diet, don't now go overboard with the vitamin tablets. It's just as bad to have a surfeit of vitamins as it is a deficit. During a harsh expedition in 1912, Antarctic explorer Xavier Mertz was forced to eat raw livers of his dogs to keep himself alive. As a consequence he died of vitamin A poisoning instead, which resulted in his skin completely peeling away from the whole of his body.) Too little essential fatty acid causes dry, scaly skin at the mild end, and in severe cases can result in serious neurological complaints. At least 15–25 grams of fat (150–250 calories) per day are needed for a healthy diet. Also, very low cholesterol is now associated with depression and violent death. At the very least, extremely low-fat diets, by depriving you of most culinary pleasures, turn out about as interesting as a party political broadcast. After all, there's a huge difference between heaps of rabbit food dressed with lemon juice (give it two days) or a civilized salad finished off with a garlicky olive oil dressing, which might just persuade you to change your eating habits permanently and save you from looking haggard. On top of everything, on very-low-fat diets hunger returns quickly, so that they have the *highest* failure rate of unbalanced diets. It's important to remember what most very-low-fat diets fail to acknowledge, namely that not all fats are bad. Indeed, polyunsaturated fats (which come from vegetable sources) are critical to good health. Thus, the typical Mediterranean diet is very high in polyunsaturated fats, especially olive oil, and, as Gilly Smith points out in *The Mediterranean Health Diet*, the population has a very low incidence of heart disease. It is only saturated fats (which come from animal sources) that have been linked to heart disease.

High-Fat Diets: Popular in the 1960s under the slogan 'eat fat and grow slim', high-fat diets have now, quite rightly, gone out of fashion since heart disease and cholesterol have become such big health issues. The first such fat diet was proposed by Hippocrates, a Greek doctor born around 460 BC and generally awarded the title of 'The Father of Medicine'. He wanted his patients to eat sesame-flavoured fatty foods once a day immediately after vigorous exercise, take *no* baths, sleep on a hard bed, and walk around naked for as long as possible. (This last perversity might be based on an understanding that the body uses more calories when cold, and thus is reminiscent of Judith Wills' *High Speed Diet*.) The main difference between this dieting oddity and the quack and fad diets of today is that Hippocrates' plan had a rather longer shelf life. Whereas now diets come and go with such rapidity that anything lasting more than a year or two is regarded as having staying power, he was on the medical bestseller lists for well over a thousand years.

A more recent version of the high-fat approach is Michel Montignac's *Eat Yourself Slim* (up to 70 per cent of calories come from fat, which makes it ironic that one of Conley's early attempts to break into the market had the same title). It introduces as its novelty factor something called the Glycemic Index, which divides carbohydrates into good and bad. His business acumen puts Rosemary Conley Enterprises to shame. 'La Galaxie Montignac' includes a chain of food shops, a 250-seat restaurant, a vineyard producing 'Château Michel Montignac', a mail-order business selling Montignac chocolate and Montignac foie gras, organizes dieting seminars for company executives at around £250 a head and runs Caribbean cruises for 'gastronomic dieters'. This diet has certainly worked for him: his various commercial ventures based on these ideas was expected to take in around £7 million in sales in 1993.

The idea behind high-fat diets is that since fat contains much of food's flavour and takes a comparatively long time to digest (it spends about three and a half hours in the stomach), the dieter should feel full for longer on pleasant food. However, in order to make sure that the food isn't too tasty, such diets tend not to permit any carbohydrates at all. No pasta dishes, no sugar, no sweet creamy desserts, no bread and little fibre. Just as many eggs, fry-ups, meat, butter and pure cream as you can get down. Is it any wonder that after a while you start to go off your food?

Low-Protein Diets: These are not to be trusted. There are few diets that make the elimination of protein the central principle of their plan (one early version was devised in Göttingen in the 1880s), but a number of the more batty proposals, by virtue of making you eat only salads or only fruits, also dangerously reduce protein intake as a consequence. So beware of any plans that cut out not just meat, fish and dairy produce, but also the good vegetable protein sources such as beans, nuts, pulses and potatoes. Human beings (in case you haven't noticed) are not caterpillars or fruitbats.

The more extreme high-fibre diets also tend to be low in protein. But human beings aren't a type of fibre-mould either. Without proteins in the diet, the body must once again turn to muscle tissue to provide the compounds (not glycogen this time, but essential amino acids) it requires for more vital processes like digestion and the production of antibodies for the immune system.

High-Protein Diets: Remember William Banting from Chapter 1, the London undertaker who gave his name to dieting? His publication *Letter on Corpulence*, the first popular diet book ever written, proposed a high-protein plan. Daily he ate 20–26 oz of meat, poultry or fish, 5–6 oz of bread or biscuit, 4–6 oz of fruit, 2 large cups of tea (without milk or sugar) and vegetables at his discretion. Low on carbohydrates, and very high on meat and fish, the best thing about this diet was that it also demanded he drink between four and six glasses of good red wine, sherry or Madeira per day. These were the days before calorie counting: depending on exactly what he ate and how he cooked it, this menu could provide anything between 1000 and 6000 calories!

In the nineteenth century, Dr James M. Salisbury invented the American Salisbury Steak, claiming that the ideal food for good health was 'the muscle pulp of lean beef made into cakes and broiled' and hot water.

High-protein diets are often, by force of circumstance, very low in carbohydrates, with all the attendant medical risks. They also tend to be high in fats and cholesterol, because red meats contain a lot of fat within the tissue, even if you cut off the fat you can see. High-protein diets should not be used by people with gout, diabetes, kidney or liver disease, or by pregnant women.

Type Four: Psychological And Spiritual Diets

Diet books that teach you to 'face up to your eating problem, give up dieting and learn to love yourself as you really are' have proliferated at a great rate since the Seventies, particularly in America. Such books usually mean well. The trouble is, they're pretty heavy going, sometimes inane. Without menus, weight loss charts or photos of women with their legs waving about in the air, it's continuous – usually humourless – text from cover to cover. There are some notable exceptions, however.

Susie Orbach's *Fat is a Feminist Issue* was truly groundbreaking. Note that it is *not* about how we should all give up dieting and learn to be happy with our weight and not subject to the patriarchial slimming industry. Her book is for compulsive eaters, and is advertised as a slimming book: the subtitle is 'how to lose weight permanently – without dieting'. Her argument, roughly speaking, is that women who eat compulsively do so because they are protesting about being sex objects – possibly true sometimes, but too sweeping and too simplistic in general.

Basically, Orbach's book is for people with eating disorders: anorexic, bulimic, thin-as-a-rake, normal-sized and large. As such, it is a very good, provocative book. It's not so much about fat as about food, and might have been entitled *Food is a Feminist Issue*. Her plan will 'teach' you how to stop hiding behind your shape, set up group therapy sessions, and, if you're overweight, talk away the fat. In the latest edition, I note, the subtitle has disappeared off the front cover, though it still remains on the title page.

Susan Kano's *Never Diet Again* is a self-help programme to teach you to love your body, break out of the dieting trap, not be taken in by media images of slenderness, etc. All good, sound, well-intentioned, well-researched stuff. Personally, when I read chapter titles like 'Learning to Love Ourselves' I want to cringe and hide in a dark cupboard, but that's an occupational hazard with psychological approaches. However, I admire Kano for having first published this book herself: that takes courage and conviction. I do wonder why, however, after all those pages against the diet industry and slimming obsession, she allowed a cover photo of a size 10, firm and just-the-fashionable-amount-of-muscle-to-fat-ratio young woman (no clue as to whether it's her or not) leaping wildly into the air. The text is relieved by some nice little illustrations – my favourite is the completely unexplained picture on page sixty of a young woman shaking hands with a genial-looking 6 ft potato.

Eve Brock's *Think Slim* ('revolutionary new approach') is one of the most daunting diet books I've yet come across, for sheer volume of information to be taken in. If only she'd had a slashing editor and different layout artist to work on it. It represents a new breed of books that hope to combine the old strict set of diet rules and menu plans with a heap of fashionable advice on how to prepare yourself psychologically for the nasty business. The idea seems clear: think positively and truthfully about yourself and you'll eliminate the excuses and acquire the motivation to get slim. And rather slim advice it turns out to be, for the most part. After you've read the 230 pages of 'Seven Steps to Slim-Fitness', identified your 'Negative Wizards', made some 'Think Slim Prompt Cards' and accepted that you're beginning a 'Lifestyle for a Lifetime', she starts you on her diet. After all that, it's just a 1000-calorie-a-day basic plan to which she allows you to add 'a little of what you fancy'. Thanks, Eve.

Another hot American import is Susan Powter's *Stop The Insanity!* You'll all know her by now: she's a close-cropped, bleached-hair dynamo, a skinhead Amazon, just bursting to tell you all about her marital problems and how they screwed her up, made her fat, made her lose her self-esteem and how she, yeah, dammit, kicked the ass off of that attitude. Motivation, I feel, is her intention. She writes staccato fashion, with lots of jabs and sentences like 'It's time to live'. Mind-blowing. I admire her independent defiance, her gutsy feminism and her scathing reference to irksome men 'with their little willies'; but I find the book astonishingly self-obsessed and – yes – plain boring: 350 pages is just too long for what she has to say. She's one of those people who can't believe that everything they do and think isn't the most fascinating stuff you'll ever hear. Oh, yes, I almost forgot: her slimming plan is eat less fat (though eat as much of everything else as you like) and exercise.

Now, on to spiritual diets. These all have delightful titles: *Help*

Lord – The Devil Wants Me Fat!, *More of Jesus and Less of Me* and *Pray Yourself Away*, written by the humorously named Charlie W. Shedd. Needless to say, they have all been big sellers in the USA. They are, in book form, a sort of cosmic version of Weight Watchers and, if you are of an evangelical turn of mind, are no doubt quite inspiring. They have yet to achieve much success in less God-fearing countries.

Slimming Clubs

Slimming clubs aim to provide motivation and a sense of shared purpose. For this reason they have some successes for those who remain with them. And, of course, their aggressive publicity campaigns make sure that the successes are very well publicized. You should remember that however impressive the weight loss stories seem, they are of little value unless we know the number of dieters who join the clubs and fail, and whether the successful slimmers *keep* the weight off. The general opinion among experts is that in the huge majority of cases they don't. Clubs are suspiciously reluctant to disclose figures, but I personally can call to mind fifteen or twenty friends who have tried them and had only the most temporary weight loss – if any at all. One American study found that 70 per cent of Weight Watchers' participants dropped out within twelve weeks. Another came up with the following mixed conclusion:

> in a 15-month follow-up study of 721 members, 50% were within 5% or less of their goal. In another study done 15 months after members had reached goal, almost 25% were below recommended weight, 46% were within 10% of goal, and 29% were 11% or more above goal.
>
> Rosenblatt, 1988

Not bad short-term success figures, but a high drop-out rate and a worryingly large proportion of dieters getting carried away into unhealthy extremes of skinniness.

When I joined Weight Watchers I found the much vaunted 'friendly atmosphere' greatly overrated. It took the best part of an hour for everybody to be weighed, during which maddeningly lacklustre period the class sat despondently around doing nothing.

The weekly lecture on food was not only the most crashingly boring affair (twenty minutes on whether to eat an apple or a piece of crispbread) but it encouraged one to go from being mildly concerned about food to being stupidly obsessive, for which luxury you paid each week, whether you attended or not. I hated it, but in fairness I must add that my aunt found her local branch very encouraging and she lost 5 st over six months. But slimming clubs do nothing to help women to feel good about themselves whatever size they are. And that is so important, if for no better reason than that a relaxed, happy person is much more likely to eat normally.

I still receive several personally addressed letters urging me to come back, together with colour photographs of 'successful slimmers'. Oddly enough, some look significantly older than before they'd slimmed. Another worrying trend I notice in diet club 'before' and 'after' photos is that the 'before' photos are getting thinner. I've seen several which showed healthy, attractively curvaceous women who were by no reasonable standard *fat*.

Weight-Control Paraphernalia

There are some marvellous objects to be put under this heading. A machine available in America counts each bite of food, and once you go over a certain number, a bell rings. You can also buy tapes that tell you how ugly you look, or a fork that lights up when there's too much food on it. There are a variety of curious clothing items that are 'guaranteed' to make you lose fat: how about a plastic 'metabolic suit' which you fill up with ice every day before putting it on, or a pair of 'Vacu-pants' which connect to the vacuum cleaner to suck away fat? There's also a claim that by suspending yourself upside down from a crossbar, 'the calories will rush to your head so they won't be absorbed in your intestine'. A blanket that 'melts your fat away while you sleep' and a whip so that you might flagellate yourself, thus stimulating the blood and carrying off fat. And so the list goes on and on and on ...

My favourite 'paraphernalia' suggestion was, however, confided to me by a lady who wrote, 'Many years ago when I wanted to lose weight, every time I felt hungry I would clean my teeth – I lost half a stone.'

If you've come across, or have invented, any others, tell me, so that I can include them in a later edition.

Drugs, Pills and Potions

Any benefit that may be produced by slimming drugs is very short lasting . . . The risks of using them far outweigh any possible benefit and they should not be used.

Professor Parish, *Medical Treatments*

The *successful* diet pill is like the aphrodisiac: vigorously sought after, often pronounced discovered, yet still unknown. There have been some marvellous suggestions in the past, and human inventiveness continues to pour forth more proposals almost by the day. All manner of rubbish has been swallowed in the earnest belief it will help women start shedding the pounds like there's no tomorrow, while the mischievous character who sold it is quietly depositing his profits in the bank and booking a flight to Honolulu.

One of the best ways of setting yourself up as a diet-pill producer is to watch the medical journals. You're sure to find soon a report on a new drug that has weight loss as a side effect, if only because it makes the user feel so sick that the very thought of food becomes repulsive. Observers noticed that Phytolacca or pokeberry reduced weight in plump migrating birds, so in 1910 a diet pill called Phytoline was put on the market. The packet burbled that it stimulated 'vital cellular physiological action' and, in complete contradiction to all scientific understanding, upgraded tissue to muscle. It also contained caffeine, a stimulant popular in such concoctions, and, just for ghoulish good measure, a touch of strychnine and arsenic.

The next step for the would-be millionaire is to hire a compressing machine and a set of pill moulds, then bung in your exotic ingredient at one end and give the result a fancy name. 'Bai-lin Tea', for example, is just a typical semi-fermented Taiwanese tea that Slimweight UK pressure-moulded into a little tablet. It doesn't do the slightest bit of good. In fact so many people complained about this one that Esther Ranzen started a campaign against it, and duly appeared, most surprisingly, as a co-author on a scientific paper published in *The Lancet* which concluded that it was a load of hooey. Numerous diet pills, potions and bath powders in the past have used citric acid on the grounds that something sour simply must be anti-fat, and I remember in my teens convincing myself that I could *feel* the nasty acidic grapefruit burning up my fat cells. Nowadays, grown canny about such marketing ploys, when

180

we see a new slimming pill advertised in glossy magazines or in the dingy back-page columns of the Sunday papers, most of us know that it's as dodgy as can be. Of course we do. But we still send off our money *just in case*. Pineapple is the current wow fruit, I hear. In the seventeenth century it was believed that fat could be reduced by rubbing on vinegar, fuller's earth, white lead, herbane juice and myrtle oil. We have not advanced since then. People around the world still get conned daily into believing that you can massage away fat, or inject water to dissolve it. Be thankful it's just a con. If it were true, and even a small fraction of the mobilized fat got into your blood stream, there would be medical hell to pay.

Appetite suppressants are often sugar-based. Since the body measures hunger by the level of sugar in the blood, these pills, which are really nothing more than a boiled sweet in tablet form, give it a temporary boost. After the boost, you'll often find that you're hungrier than ever. A more worrying constituent of diet pills in the early part of the century was dinitrophenol, better known during World War I as the main constituent of certain explosives, and listed as an industrial toxin since 1889. The pill was suppressed in 1938.

A more straightforward diet 'aid' is a packet of little rubber pellets that are shaped like maggots. Sprinkle them on your food, and behold! You won't want to eat it. I expect it won't be long before someone starts marketing real maggots: far more effective!

Now let's look at the more serious drugs. My chief reference work has been Peter Parish's *Medicines: A Guide for Everybody.*

Amphetamines and their Relatives: In the Fifties and Sixties doctors prescribed billions of amphetamines ('speed') for their stimulant and appetite-suppressing effect. Come the Seventies there was a dramatic reduction in sales after the serious mental consequences of long-term use were realized, including delirium, paranoid hallucinations and delusions, and panic states, leading to possible suicidal and homicidal urges, and in some cases permanent mental breakdown. Having been prescribed amphetamines myself I can vouch for the fact that they seriously wind you up – after a few days I felt a nervous, shaking wreck. I also found they ruined my complexion: I remember looking in the mirror and seeing a grey, drained face stare back at me. Among their more enduring side effects are liver damage, high blood pressure and bleeding into the brain.

Some doctors still prescribe amphetamine-related drugs, including *diethylpropion* (Apisate and Tenuate Dospan), *phentermine* (Duromine and Ionamin) for prolonged periods of weight loss, even though it is now well known that the reduction in appetite lasts only a few weeks. My advice is: stay away from them; they'll create more problems than they cure.

Fenfluramine (Ponderax) is another amphetamine-related drug, though not a stimulant. It increases the concentration of serotonin, a stimulant chemical in the brain, which in turn makes you feel full. Back in the Seventies I was prescribed Ponderax for slimming and experienced terrifying mental symptoms that lasted for days: panic, disorientation and depersonalization. *Dexfenfluramine* (Adifax) is similar to Ponderax.

Diuretics: These are popular slimming tablets in spite of the fact that they have no impact on fat at all. They are dehydrating drugs, temporarily reducing your *weight* (not fat) by making you go to the loo more often. As soon as you stop taking them, your kidneys will stop passing urine until your water level has returned to normal. A low-salt diet will do the same sort of thing, and, in most diets, the high initial weight loss that you see whatever diet you are following can usually be attributed to water loss rather than anything more substantial.

Bulk Foods and Laxatives (e.g. Celevac, Cellucon, Guarem, Nilstim, Prefil): These usually contain non-digestible plant substances which swell up in either the stomach (thereby reducing your appetite by making you feel full, though the sensation lasts only for half an hour or so) or the bowels (increasing the size and absorbency of your stools). They work in the same way as diuretics, by dehydration, and have no impact at all on fat. As with diuretics, as soon as you stop using them your water content and weight go back to what they were. Part of the trouble is the bulking fibre used in these preparations. If soluble fibre (such as beans and oats) were used instead they'd probably be a bit more effective. The only difficulty is that soluble fibre causes flatulence. If you want to fill up with few calories before a meal it's much easier and cheaper to eat carrots or an apple; and if you're determined to take laxatives, it's tastier to eat prunes.

Herbal Remedies: These usually use either bulking agents or diuretics. Unfortunately, there's recently been some difficulty with these types of pills because some of the ingredients have turned out to be poisonous. So approach them with caution.

Thyroid Drugs: These first became common in the late 1920s. They work by increasing your metabolic rate and can lead to fever, vomiting, angina, disordered heart beat, osteoporosis, sudden death (when overdosed), and so on. They 'should never be used as an aid to slimming' says Dr Parish, though, alas, they too often are. Between 60 and 80 per cent of the weight lost is lean tissue, not fat, and there's rapid weight regain after treatment, perhaps because the thyroid supplement has reduced the function of the slimmer's own thyroid. Even in doses far below those used for slimming, these pills have been shown to increase mortality by over 20 per cent. It's even worse when thyroid pills are combined with anorectic agents like amphetamines, which is common practice.

Cocaine: The Indians of the Andes chew coca leaf to stop themselves feeling hungry. Benzocaine, which works by numbing the tongue, is supposed to have a similar effect, but only in the short term. Cocaine is not only illegal, but use can lead to extremely unpleasant mental disturbance, paranoia, and physical side effects. The reputation of cocaine as a relatively safe, trendy jet-set drug is highly misleading. It can be deadly.

Starch Blockers: These pills work by preventing the digestion of starch in the intestine, which results in malnutrition. They are made from a protein found in red kidney beans. Some of the more slap-dash preparations contained just ground-up kidney beans.

Sorry to be such a killjoy, but the truth is that diet pills are usually a waste of money. In fact, money's about the only thing they've got going for them, because, if you pay enough for a pill, then you are so determined to get value that you often end up going on a severe diet as well just to ensure success. The late A. T. W. Simeons charged hundreds of dollars for his six-week course of injections of a 'brilliant' new slimming compound known as Human Chorionic Gonadotropin (HCG). How could something with such a name not work? You had also, of course, to go on a 500-calorie-a-day diet. And, surprise, surprise, after a while you lost weight! And who was to know that HCG was really a compound obtained from pregnant women's urine?

Having read this chapter I hope you are beginning to see just

how pointless, and indeed repetitive, these endless diet preparations are. The main value of a good diet book is to provide
sensible *guidelines* on what to eat, and, more importantly, morale
and motivation. If there's a writer who really does fire you with
enthusiasm to adopt a reasonable eating pattern, all well and good.
Otherwise you'd do far better to turn to Part Three and aim for
your own healthy-eating plan.

But just in case you do stumble upon some marvellous dieting
method that succeeds beyond your wildest dreams and you
become too thin, let's give the last word to the Toilet Specialist:

> The best mode of treatment for a 'scraggy' – horrible, though
> expressive word – person would be a term of incarceration in
> an Eastern harem; but this is, of course, out of the question.
>
> 'Early to bed and early to rise' should be parodied to
> 'Early to bed and *late* to rise' in the case of everyone who
> desires to get plump. Lie in bed as long as you can. The
> very best diet is one exclusively composed of fish, eggs,
> milk, soups, vegetables, farinaceous food, grains, fruits, and
> sweets. All acids should be avoided, whether drinks or meals;
> sugary and oily forms of food should be given the distinct
> preference. Vinegar, of course, should not be used in *any*
> form; salt only sparingly; mustard may, however, be eaten
> freely.
>
> Singing is good for all women; it helps to pass a larger
> quantity of fresh air than usual in the chest and lungs, and
> the walls of the former are thereby made more elastic, with
> a consequent additional nutrition of the tissues.

So there you are. Skinnies, get singing!

10

Drastic Measures

Surgical and Other Non-dietary Methods of Changing Your Figure

I suspect you're going to read this chapter with the same ghoulish curiosity with which I began researching it.

Having seen in the previous chapter how very inadequate, often downright dangerous, so many diets are, you may wonder whether there are more successful ways of shedding flesh. I've tried in what follows to give a good idea of the most important techniques. It's a rapidly changing field, however, and new methods are being developed all the time. So, as with the Diet Digest, this is only an indication of what's available, not an exhaustive list.

There are various ways of interfering with the body: I'll begin at the mouth, and move downwards.

Jaw Wiring: Not only the most well-known, but also the most straightforward of such methods, jaw wiring is exactly what it sounds like: a way to clamp the mouth shut and thus physically prevent too much food from being put in. After a thorough dental checkup to ensure that there are no problems likely to erupt suddenly, thin wires are passed between your teeth and twisted together. You must then exist on liquid food, taken through a straw. Sounds simple? It does have certain disadvantages. Aside from the indignity of being made to feel like a medieval torture victim, the wires soon start to rub on your gums and lips, leading possibly to ulcers. You may also suffer painful spasms of your jaw. To avoid some of the abrasive complications caused by so much wire, an alternative approach is to cast two stainless steel covers, one for the upper and one for the lower jaw, and then cement them in place and wire them together. This gives you a better chance of making it in a James Bond screen test, but prevents you speaking, laughing, brushing your teeth and vomiting. Very smelly, and rather scary. Hettie:

> I could only talk through gritted teeth and this gave me a permanent headache. My jaw ached so much I could have cried. Worst of all I was terrified that I would be sick – it's very easy to suffocate or choke on your own vomit.

Karen made a different point:

> In a way you're only swapping one kind of difficulty for another. Yes, I lost weight, but I went through agonies – and I mean agonies – of longing for food. I was like a heroin addict confronted with piles of the drug yet unable to sample any. This made me really panic. Having gone through all that I actually find it less stressful to force myself to do without.

However, for those whose weight is debilitating, or needs to be lost for surgery, obviously some method is required if all dietary approaches fail, and this one has the benefit of being non-invasive. Overall it is comparatively low-risk and as effective as any of the surgical methods. The trouble, as with all rapid-weight-loss techniques, is that the weight rapidly comes back on again afterwards. It was in an effort to counteract this that the following device was invented:

The Waist Cord: The simplest approach. A nylon cord, its ends fused or knotted together, encircles the patient's waist. If your girth increases, the cord cuts into you. The idea is that after a couple of agonizingly big meals you are forced into the habit of eating less and keeping off the weight you have lost through jaw wiring. Of course, it is always possible, and sometimes necessary (in the case of, for example, fluid retention during your period), to cut the cord, but on the whole the technique has been quite successful in keeping down weight regain after drastic loss, at least in the short term. I've found that my own version of this – namely a close-fitting pair of jeans – is a good way to keep weight off. It only requires that you wear the jeans every couple of days. Then, as soon as they get to feel uncomfortable, cut down on what you eat. Invariably my weight creeps up when I start wearing loose garments, when I conveniently forget about my expanding girth.

Next stop, the stomach (there's no point chopping around the oesophagus, because nothing gets absorbed there). We are now into the arena of . . .

Surgical Techniques: Most of these are seriously risky, and are supposed to be used only for patients with 'refractory morbid obesity', the definition of which term depends on whose surgery you attend. The general guidelines are that the patient should be between eighteen and fifty years old, and for ten years or more at least 100 per cent or 100 lbs above her recommended weight, during which period all other non-surgical methods should have been tried. However, after these methods first became popular in the Seventies, 'the criteria for acceptance became looser and looser until now anyone who is even moderately plump can find a cooperative surgeon', according to the American magazine *Radiance*. Since the severely obese are thought to be anaesthetic risks (although there is some doubt about whether this is true or not), jaw wiring is often used as a way of reducing the weight in order to allow the next stage, namely stomach-stapling, to take place.

(a) **Stomach Stapling:** This is where you can let your imagination wander. Think of it as a GCSE question. You have just been handed a stomach (which is a thing shaped rather like an enormous kidney bean, with the food dropping in from the top and passing out at the bottom). Your objective is to reduce it from its usual capacity of about two pints, down to just over the size of a single shot of whisky from the pub (and we all know how small that is). The food must, on its travels, be allowed a good dousing of digestive fluids. You have at your disposal one staple gun filled with stainless steel staples, a needle and thread, a sharp knife and, should you decide to get fancy . . . anything else you care to mention.

Once you get the hang of the idea, you can see there is a whole host of possibilities. So go on, get out a piece of paper and pencil and see how you might go about it (there's a fortune in it if you have a real brainwave).

Here are some solutions provided by the surgeons:
(i) The simplest approach is horizontal gastroplasty, or dividing the stomach horizontally with a line of staples, leaving only a small connecting gap of about a centimetre. The food coming down the oesophagus, instead of plunging into a nice big stomach at

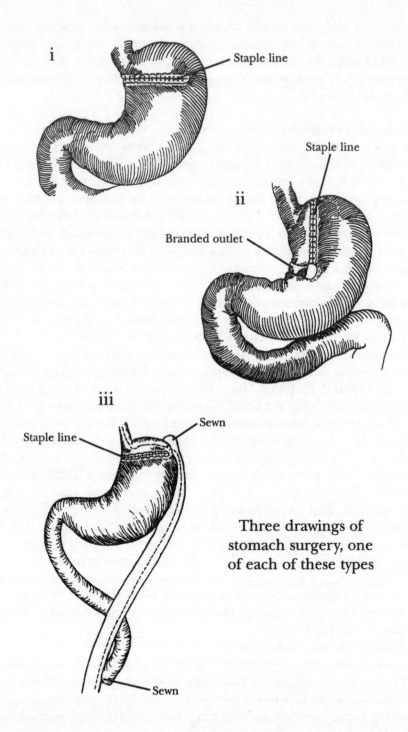

i — Staple line

ii — Staple line

Branded outlet

iii — Staple line — Sewn

Sewn

Three drawings of
stomach surgery, one
of each of these types

the end, finds itself crammed into a tiny first stomach, through which it has to squash its way before plopping down into the larger second stomach. This means that if you eat anything more than the smallest bit of solid, the first stomach gets too full and you vomit everything back up the way it came.

(ii) Vertical banded gastroplasty is rather more complicated and takes about two hours to complete. The idea is, in effect, to staple the stomach up in such a way that the top part is unused, except for a corridor allowing the food to pass down into the bottom part. A hole is then cut into the stomach at the bottom of the staple line, allowing a band to be placed around the outlet to prevent it stretching.

(iii) Another method is to staple the top part of the stomach off completely, cut out an exit hole, then slice off and attach a bit of the intestine and bypass the bottom part of the stomach all together by attaching the other end of the piece of intestine lower down the digestive tract. The full title for this two-and-a-half- to three-hour operation is Roux-en-Y gastrojejunostomy, and it is preferred for sweet eaters, since the dumping of improperly digested sugar directly into the intestine has particularly unpleasant consequences which, it is hoped, will put you off ever eating sweets again.

But do they work? Is it really worth having some medical bloke poking about in such intimate areas, while you lie in anesthetic oblivion? The first problem with these techniques is that within a few days of stomach reduction around one in twenty-five of the patients will die from suffocation, peritonitis, and blood clots in the lungs. Other complications include bloating of the stomach pouch, nausea and vomiting. In up to 15 per cent of cases the staple line bursts open (more delicately termed 'dehiscence'), and further deaths can occur due to liver failure. Stomach cancer, immune deficiency, brain and nerve damage are also possible. If you get past these hurdles, food should be in liquid form only for the first six weeks, and thereafter solid foods are allowed provided you chew slowly and thoroughly. The benefit of the operation is counteracted if you drink calorie-dense foods like milkshakes and soft drinks.

But worst of all, once again, the beneficial effect is only short-term. Stomachs are maddeningly elastic and can extend to accommodate more food. This often results in a plateau after six to twelve months so that most patients still remain 60–80 per cent above their recommended weights. If the staples are actually removed, then the lost weight starts to come back with a vengeance, because the operation has done nothing to change your eating habits. As one woman quoted in *Woman's Own* explained:

> When I came round from the operation I felt as if I'd been ripped apart – the pain was excruciating. I'd been cut from my navel to my breasts ... Psychologically, though, I still had my old attitudes to food and I began to binge again. It stretched my staples and made me violently sick ...

This particular patient's weight went shooting up as soon as the staples were taken out. Bravely, she had the operation a second time, and lives now 'on crackers and soup. I'll have to have my stomach staples in for ever'.

Still, for people who are so large that they can't move properly (a problem most common in America, where weights of 40 st are not uncommon, and some people have been known to weigh up to 80 st) the potential risks of the operation may well be outbalanced by the enormous drawbacks of excessive weight, despite the fact that the operation is probably more likely to kill them than their bulk.

(b) **The Gastric Balloon:** In an effort to avoid the trauma of invasive surgery, some bright spark came up with the idea of inserting a deflated balloon into the stomach, via a tube, and then pumping it up to about a pint in volume. The tube is then removed, and the balloon left to float freely. By pressing against the stomach walls it is supposed to give an impression of fullness. One early patient was treated with an ordinary 'dime store balloon', but these days they are made from latex (which has a tendency to deflate after a couple of weeks) or silicone (which lasts from three to six months). Gastric ulcers, nausea, vomiting, fainting, and heartburn are all possible complaints, and obstruction of the intestine following deflation has led to some deaths. One woman speaking on Robert Kilroy Silk's BBC programme *Dying for Your Figure* explained how her stomach tried to reject the balloon. For three days she was in such pain she thought she was having a constant heart attack. The main drawback of gastric balloons, however, is that of all the radical approaches, they seem the least efficacious. One version widely used in America was found to be 'no more effective than a sham procedure in favouring weight loss'.

Oh dear.

Let's move on to the intestines . . .

(c) **Intestinal Bypass:** The intestine is what remains of the digestive tract after the food has emerged from the stomach. Further
digestion of some foods takes place here, as well as the absorption
of the broken-down molecules into the body. Normally about 20 ft
long, under general anaesthetic the intestines are sometimes
reduced to just 1 ft in length, so that only tiny amounts of food
get the proper treatment. Since you can't pull out the excluded
19 ft of gut, it is left in to hang about. You could say an intestinal
bypass is the surgical version of a laxative: it's all through you and
into the loo before you have time to say 'excess calorie'.

The mortality rate of this method is about one in twenty. Sixty
to seventy per cent of operations result in one or more of thirty-
seven possible complications ranging from liver failure to diarrhoea, the last of which occurs because so little of the food eaten
is digested. Because of the high risks, these days intestinal bypass is
reserved mainly for the most severe cases involving otherwise
untreatable weight-related illnesses, though 'improved techniques'
are gradually making it more popular again.

A further drawback is that after a year and a half the weight
loss levels off because the reduced segment of intestine gradually
adapts, becoming thicker and longer, and better at absorbing
calories.

To conclude surgical methods are not a magic answer. They
should not even be considered by anyone who is not at least
twice the recommended weight or in desperate need of substantial
weight loss for health reasons. In these cases surgery can give you
a kick start in the right direction, but unless you can succeed in
overcoming your body's physiological and psychological defences
against weight loss, the pounds will inevitably come back. The only
real answer, long term, is through changing eating habits and
reducing naturally. If you're going to have to learn new habits in
the end, why not learn them at the beginning and do without the
surgery? Remember what the patient quoted above said: 'I don't
think it's the answer – no surgery is. The answer can only come
from you.'

Cosmetic Surgery

A different way of getting rid of flesh. Even ten years ago cosmetic surgery was, in England, at least, regarded as the plaything of the Michael Jacksons of this world: rich people with nothing better to do than muck about with their bodies. Now everybody's doing it. A popular women's magazine recently photographed an average family of four who had all had something done (mostly to their perfectly normal faces). There are no end of ways in which you can have yourself interfered with, but what you must remember is that cosmetic surgery is not a weight-loss technique; it's a fashion aid. If you're a fashion victim of the particularly slavish variety, then this is the way forward.

(a) **Liposuction:** The removal of fat cells by liquidizing and sucking them out with a vacuum, this is already the most popular cosmetic operation in the United States (about 150,000 a year at the time of going to press) and is rapidly gaining ground here (about 7500 a year). Liposuction can be practised on most parts of the body: arms, breasts, thighs, ankles, buttocks, knees, abdomen and even the face, but only 5 lbs of fat at most can safely be removed, and for this to be successful the patient must be young so that the skin is sufficiently elastic to tighten over the treated areas. Once you get to your mid-forties, liposuction is not much use. At any age it's risky and very painful.

The British Association of Aesthetic Plastic Surgeons (BAAPS) warns that 'you can expect considerable bruising which will be uncomfortable and, at times, painful'. All the women I spoke to laughed when I read this to them: in each case it had been 'sheer agony', 'unbelievably unpleasant', 'excruciating', 'bloody agony'. Susan:

> I'd been counselled, but I wasn't prepared for it. I had it done at a private clinic. The surgeon had a felt-tip pen and marked me out like a piece of meat, or a paper-cutting pattern. I woke about four hours later in agony. The pain continued for hours, a deep throbbing pain all over my lower regions. I couldn't straighten my legs, they hurt so much.

Want to know what happened while Susan was asleep? The following is an eyewitness account, quoted in Naomi Wolf's *The Beauty Myth*, by American journalist Jill Neimark:

192

[A] man force[s] a plastic tube down a naked woman's throat. He connects the tube to a pump that, for the next two hours, will breathe for her. Her eyes are taped shut, her arms are stretched out horizontally and her head lolls a little to the side . . . What comes next is almost unbelievably violent. Her surgeon . . . begins to thrust the cannula in and out, as rapid as a piston, breaking through thick nests of fat nerves and tissue in her leg. The doctor is ready to stitch her up. Nearly 2,000 millilitres of tissue and blood have been sucked out of her, any more would put her at risk of massive infection and fluid loss leading to shock and death . . . He peels the tape back from her lids, and she stares at him, unseeing. 'A lot of people have trouble coming back. Bringing someone out of anaesthesia is the most dangerous part of an operation.' . . . [which] can lead to massive infection, excessive damage to capillaries and fluid depletion resulting in shock and coma.

It is not known how many people have died from liposuction. BAAPS does not keep statistics, which is unsurprising, given the profits to be made from this type of operation (£1000–£3000, depending on the part of body involved).

Cosmetic surgery is also addictive. *Newsweek* called the patients 'scalpel slaves', who 'go from doctor to doctor, seeking multiple operations . . . Their self-scrutiny becomes microscopic'. On the television programme *Hollywood Women*, the women interviewed agreed that it is easy to become addicted to the process: some visited their plastic surgeons up to once a *month*.

It's addictive two fold. If it works, you think, great, how can I improve myself next? If it doesn't work, you think, God, how can I correct this problem? Or it can be a combination of the two. I always admired my small waist, but hated my big thighs. After I had liposuction my thighs looked good, but my waist suddenly seemed disproportionately large. So I had to have that done too. In the end, my whole body was out of kilter, and I was constantly trying to get it right. All in all I don't think I actually look any better than four years and £30,000 ago.

(b) **Abdominoplasty:** The surgical removal of fat from the abdomen may have been practised even as early as Roman and Talmudic Jewish times. The first modern such surgery, then called a 'lipectomy', was reported in 1889. The name of the operation now is 'abdominoplasty', or, for those of a cute turn of mind, a 'tummy tuck'. It is a method only for tightening loose skin, slack muscles and stretch marks caused by pregnancy or rapid weight loss. In order to minimize the risks you should be at your weight on the weight chart before the operation, and if you're not, you must diet to get there. If you gain or lose weight afterwards, get pregnant again or do abdominal exercises, the effects will be lost and scars will stretch.

For the operation, which costs about £2000, you'll be cut from hip bone to hip bone more or less below the bikini line. Then the surgeon pulls the skin down from the rib cage, snips off the excess and cuts a new hole for the navel, before stitching you up again. The whole thing lasts about ninety minutes, and you will be left with permanent scars which may not, after all, says the BAAPS blithely, 'lie entirely within the confines of fashionable swimwear'. Furthermore, because 'sensory nerves are necessarily interupted [sic] when freeing the skin and fat from the muscles' (i.e., the nerves have been ripped apart as the fat is sliced away) you may also be left permanently numb in the stomach region.

After the operation (providing it works, which is not always the case) you will be hospitalized for three or four days with 'moderately severe pain' and drainage tubes emerging from each side of your stomach region to drain off blood into bottles. You will need to take things extremely easy for two weeks and have at least three weeks off work. Risks include chest infection, thrombosis and heavy bleeding, the last of which will necessitate a second operation.

(c) **Breast Adjustment:** It is one of the great female tragedies that women with bosoms hate them and women without bosoms long for them. A hundred years ago the problem was only one way: the Toilet Specialist has great sympathy with any woman suffering 'want of plumpness in her arms and bust', and she suggests as a remedy daily friction to the bosom with a concoction of linseed oil and myrrh, or a diet of black grapes.

Today we have surgical breast enlargement, but it is not a happy option. Cindy Jackson, cited earlier, who has had just about everything done to her body and talks about it on television, finally decided that her bosoms weren't big enough:

I had a 1½ in incision made underneath each breast. The

surgeon inserted his hands and made a pocket. The silicone implant was placed behind the muscle on the wall of my chest. It was then sewn up, leaving a tiny scar. It was very painful. After the operation I felt sick and my breasts felt hot and swollen – they looked like missiles. I could hardly move for days.

The results disappointed me. Once the swelling had gone down I was a 34D cup, but that didn't feel big enough. Three months later the left breast became hard and painful. Scar tissue was forming round the implant. Surgeons broke it free by twisting it – it was agony. Half of the implant then slipped behind the muscle, making my breasts uneven . . .

Woman

In up to seven out of ten cases the operation results in hardened scar tissue around the implant and the breasts have to be reopened and the implants ripped out. The implants can be either saltwater or silicone: both leak, the second resulting possibly in immune-system dysfunction and toxic shock syndrome. While implants do not appear to cause cancer, they make it much harder to detect it, with the result that many women will die from a terrifying disease that might, given earlier warning, have been cured. Any operation on the breast may also result in permanent desensitizing of the nipple to some degree, and possibly the death of it, though – again, unsurprisingly – this drawback is invariably underplayed in the promotional literature. Furthermore, the implant will be readily detected on touch and, because it is a separate item from the mammary tissue, will show, by distorting the outline of your breast, whenever you move too vigorously.

I have more sympathy with breast *reduction* because a very large bosom can cause no end of trouble. Jenny:

I've had continual pain in my neck and shoulders and my posture's suffered because of the weight of my breasts. My bra straps dig into my skin and I've even had rashes because of sweat collecting down between the breasts.

In addition to permanent pain and discomfort, women with large breasts endure sniggers and jibes from other people. Katie Boyle, who's had the operation, has spoken most eloquently of the nuisance of enormous boobs, not least of which is the difficulty of turning over in bed at night!

But once again it is not an operation to be considered lightly. Jenny's cost her £3500. She was three hours on the operating table, during which time her nipples were cut away with what some surgeons like to term a 'cookie cutter', and replaced. She has permanent scarring and a one-in-five chance that the nipple will become necrotic and drop off.

Is It Really Worth It?

Surgery for drastic weight loss is dangerous, debilitating, often appallingly painful and, perhaps most significant of all, is rarely effective in the long term. But for some people (far fewer than actually have such operations) it does appear to be the only resort.

Cosmetic surgery, on the other hand, is usually more of a psychological treatment than a physical one. The pressure on people – women in particular – to give up their individuality and conform to a mass-marketed image of beauty and bland normality has become so great that it's unsurprising how many buckle under it. Magazines run regular features on women who have endured one or another cosmetic agony and exclaim they are delighted with the results and would do the whole thing over again if need be, without hesitation. Many women, in this supposedly emancipated age, have become so obsessive about even the minutest details of their figures that, short of a cultural U-turn, it seems as if cosmetic surgery is the only means left of giving them at least temporary peace of mind. For what it's worth, they have my sympathy. But let me point out that those magazine articles usually paint a very rosy picture of what is, in fact, a very dark subject.

So, if you feel inclined, my advice is: don't do it. People won't admire you more for it; men probably won't notice the difference; the risks of scarring and worse are great; the market is full of charlatans who could seriously ruin your looks altogether; the pain can be extraordinary; and, though it may provide a boost at first, it only contributes in the end to the rotting away of your self-esteem. You'd make yourself far more lovable by spending the money on something that contributed to your soul: £2000 will take you on a trip round China, or buy you a small car for independence, give you flying lessons, teach you to ski or sail, allow you to do something you've always dreamed of.

We should have enough self-respect not to pay surgeons to chop us painfully around as if we were living several hundred years ago and our whole value rested on our looks. I agree with actor Lenny Henry who, when asked by *Woman* magazine if he would have cosmetic surgery, replied:

> Get out of here! That's for neurotic, lazy people who'd rather have fat sucked out of their butts than go to a gym and do something about it. Nose jobs are for losers, too – people who don't realize that a nose job changes your nose, not your life.

Okay, he's a man and there aren't the same pressures to be beautiful. But more and more men are going in for surgery – even such ridiculous things as calf implants (how far can vanity go?). It is vital that we do not give in to such pressures. When you opt for cosmetic surgery it is not a private decision: you are upping the stakes for all women and pandering to the ridiculous notion that we ought to be perfect. After our hard-won emancipation we should be fighting ideas like this, not giving in to them. I do agree with the following letter, sent by a reader to *Woman* magazine:

> We were watching a TV programme about Hollywood women having cosmetic surgery, when I said to my husband about one of them, 'She does look prettier, doesn't she?' 'I suppose so,' he said, 'but for me she looks exactly the same as all the others now.'

Nevertheless, if you're dead set on cosmetic surgery, at least consider the matter carefully for three or four months. Spend the interval exercising, seeing a decent (female) counsellor, researching the true risks (not tame versions announced in the promotional literature) and reading books by the likes of Shelley Bovey, Germaine Greer and Naomi Wolf. Never, never, never agree to surgery because your partner is putting pressure on you. Any man who does this is unequivocally a *C-R-E-E-P.* (Try insisting he has an operation to make his penis larger.)

If, after that, you are still determined, then for heaven's sake go to someone reputable. Best of all, visit several surgeons and compare what they say. Ask to be put in touch with former patients. One woman I spoke to received alarmingly conflicting advice when she shopped around. Never trust a surgeon who encourages you to do more than you are happy with – anybody reputable will, if anything, point out the disadvantages. There are an increasing number of malpractice suits in cosmetic surgery. Cindy Jackson, whom I referred to earlier as having undergone major plastic surgery all over her body in order to achieve the look she favoured, has now set up an independent consumer organization called the Cosmetic Surgery Network at P.O. Box 3410, London N6 4EE. 'I tell patients what really works and what doesn't ... I'd say that only five or six of the 200 surgeons practising cosmetic surgery in the country know what they are doing,' she told the *Independent on Sunday.* So be really tough: it's you who are going to have to live with the consequences.

11

Slimming or Starving?

To maintain hunger where food is available, as Western women are doing, is to submit to a life state as unnatural as anything with which the species has come up yet. It is more bizarre than cannibalism.

Naomi Wolf

Jean Ross, a 5 ft 7 ins caterer, was on a 1200-calorie-a-day diet. After eight days she could no longer bear it and hurried out in her lunch hour and bought three bars of chocolate. Half an hour later she was full of guilt and self-disgust: 'God I'm such a pig, a greedy revolting pig!'

Two weeks before, she had helped organize a university reunion dinner, at which 200 former students got together and happily munched their way through six courses: starting with mushroom tartlets and Hollandaise sauce, and ending on Pavlova. If Jean, on 1200 calories, was a 'revolting pig', it would be difficult to find a name appropriate to these greedy scoffers: super dinosaur-sized pigs, perhaps? 'Oh no,' said Jean, shocked. 'That's different. They're men for one thing.'

Guilt and self-disgust are integral parts of dieting. One of the reasons the dieting industry goes from strength to strength is that dieters always blame themselves, not the diet. Is there another product under the sun which, if it failed *once*, never mind time and time again, we would continue to pay good money for? Of course not. So it is high time that we turned things the right way up: Jean Ross was not 'a pig' because she could not stick to 1200 calories. She is not weak-willed and self-indulgent. It is the diets themselves that are utterly unreasonable. Our responses to them are quite normal, healthy and, indeed, often exceedingly brave.

1000 Calories a Day Is Not Enough!

During all the many years when I was dieting – whether following a particular regime or simply counting my own calories – the standard wisdom was this: approximately 2000 calories per day are necessary for an average woman to function, therefore 1000 calories was a reasonable dieting allowance. We all know what a ludicrous amount of food you get for 1000 calories: if you actually bother to weigh and measure it you're always astonished at the tiny little portions. Go just a wee bit over and the calories start shooting up. But, even if your partner is sympathetic, we get little reassurance from the doctors and slimming clubs: 'Now, now, don't be greedy!' they admonish. 'No willpower, that's your trouble. Anyone would think you were starving.'

How right they are. 1000 calories a day *is* a semi-starvation diet. Let's make some comparisons.

India is one of the poorest countries in the world. I have been there many times, toured the country from top to toe, seen the huge range of incomes, lifestyles, castes, figures, from the beautifully voluptuous Sikh ladies to the small, skeletal women bringing up little scraps of children. Here, the very poorest women, probably rarely taller than 5 ft 4 ins and often substantially smaller, eat how much?

1400 Calories a Day

We all know something – vaguely – about the peasants of olden days. Poverty was rife: the rich stuffed themselves while the poor half-starved. So how many calories would a fifteenth-century peasant actually consume?

3200 Calories a Day

Of course, in those days people took considerably more exercise, but they were also shorter and therefore probably had lower calorie requirements in the first place. Even allowing for our more sedentary lifestyle, noting that the biggest slice of one's daily calorie requirements is just for keeping the body alive, let alone kicking, makes it clear that 1000 calories a day is dangerously low.

The great Dutch famine began in May 1940, during the German occupation of the Netherlands. The Dutch authorities, apportioning rations, established the level of semi-starvation as between 600 and 1600 calories per day. Once a person had lost 25 per cent of her body weight, she was considered to be 'starving' and so entitled to precious supplements. Naomi Wolf, commenting on photographs of Dutch women of the period, remarks 'how preternaturally modern they look'. At Treblinka concentration camp, 900 calories were determined to be the minimum necessary to sustain human functioning.

These statistics – and scores like them – give a rather different complexion to our attempts to diet. Many modern regimes insist on daily calorie allowances far lower than 1000. Whether the semi-starvation is self-inflicted or inflicted by famine or Nazis, the effects are the same: anxiety, depression, fatigue, irritability, poor concentration, lassitude, slowed metabolism, social isolation and, of course, an overriding obsession with food. After years of dieting I have now stopped, but I still get slightly nervous when I go out to dinner and see that the hostess has not provided quite as much food as seems necessary for all the guests. If I am handed a portion that is smaller than my neighbour's I am filled with irrational fury. I abominate most the hostess who, surveying some delicious looking remains in the casserole dish on the table, whisks it from under the diners' noses saying, 'Mmmm, that'll do nicely for lunch tomorrow.' These reactions of mine always seemed so greedy and ignominious, until I read that dieting is widely known to induce the sort of behaviour also seen in orphans adopted from poor countries, who continue to smuggle and hide food for years after it has become plentiful.

A recent article in the *Independent on Sunday* entitled 'Serves one (ha ha)', on ready-prepared meals, including diet foods, had everyone agreeing on their feeble quantities:

> 'I can easily shovel down two Lean Cuisines at one go, and frequently do. With extra garlic bread on the side,' confesses Amanda, a solicitor. 'Mean Cuisine, more like,' she added crossly.

Another tester, having demolished a Bird's Eye Healthy Options Chicken Tikka Masala ('Complete Balanced Meal on a Plate'), responded 'Serves one *what?*'

So, if you still insist on going on low-calorie diets, when you fail to stick to them – or indeed when you succeed, but only after painful lamentations and suffering – at least spare yourself *guilt*. These rations are pitiful.

Disordered Eating

When I began researching this book I knew that most women diet, whether they need to lose weight or not. But I was not prepared for the truly staggering number of women who (secretly) suffer some degree of disordered eating. I remember when, three or four years ago, the press (surely desperate for something sensational to invent?) announced that Princess Diana was so thin she must be anorexic. I laughed at such a ridiculous suggestion. Now we know that the press got it only slightly wrong, for Diana was bulimic, (bulimia and anorexia frequently overlap). Since these revelations the subject has had a huge amount of media coverage. But what exactly is 'disordered eating'?

'Disordered eating' refers to a continuous spectrum of unnatural eating habits: at one extreme, anorexia due to self-starvation; at the other, obesity due to constant, unstoppable eating. An anorexic is intensely afraid of gaining weight, considers herself fatter than she is, has missed at least three consecutive menstrual cycles, or is 15 per cent below her expected weight. Lord Byron, Franz Kafka and the author of *Peter Pan*, J. M. Barrie, are all now thought to have been anorexics (menstrual irregularities excepted, one assumes). Novelist Virginia Woolf became obsessive about not eating. She rebelled against what she saw as the whole disgusting process of feeding and excreting; food became a key feature in her mental illness.

Bulimia lies between the two extremes, though most such conditions are hard to characterize exactly. Broadly speaking, anorexia (from the Greek for 'no longing') involves self-starvation, and bulimia (Greek: 'ox-hunger'), a cycle of severe dieting followed by binges and then purging through excessive exercise, dieting, vomiting or laxative abuse – some bulimics swallow up to 100 laxative tablets a day. I must admit, hearing of such practices, I formed a picture of someone rather odd: a tortured adolescent, a spiky-haired punk perhaps, or a social misfit. But, looking through the literature, case history after case history features *perfectly ordinary women* with perfectly ordinary jobs, the kind of people one deals with every day: librarians, schoolteachers, housewives, shop assistants, as well as whizz-kid executives, media personalities and the like.

Bulimia has a long and distinguished history. It was diagnosed as early as the second century AD by the Greek doctor, Galen, and the term referred, for a long time, simply to people with a superlative appetite. In 1678 the case of a man was documented who 'from his youth was wont, with a strange kind of greediness, to take in all sort of food and as speedily to eject them'. Shortly after, a labourer from Stanton, Lancashire, was described as having 'ox-hunger' before the Royal Society. At each meal he was in the habit of eating a whole roast leg of veal, and for dessert he went out into the fields and consumed 'sow-thistles and divers other Herbs greedily as the Beasts who were wont to eat such food'. However, this man's trouble turned out to be 'divers Worms, as long as an ordinary Tobacco pipe', which he eventually 'voided' and then he returned to normal. It was only in 1979 that bulimia was recognized as a distinctive disorder, characterized by a cycle of bingeing and purging, guilt, fear of not being able to stop eating and, again, excessive concern about gaining weight.

Apart from the clinical extremes of anorexia and bulimia, there is a wealth of sub-clinical disordered eating patterns that are rarely discussed. For example, my own vigorous attempts to lose weight by starving all day until I felt sick, faint and dizzy and then gorging one enormous meal at night. It is estimated that at least 50 per cent of British women suffer from some type of disordered eating behaviour.

While I was researching this book, women whom I had previously assumed to be in control of every aspect of their lives started revealing their secret anguish. Charlotte, a thirty-five-year-old solicitor who is forceful, successful, extremely attractive and with a *very slim* figure, poured forth a history of disordered eating and food obsessions. She hated her body ('those horrible curves, I wish I could be like a boy'). Shelley Bovey cites Jill Welbourne, who has treated women of all sizes for a variety of emotional problems:

> 'Being thin is what kills you,' she says. And she is prepared to put herself on the line for her controversial observations, based on many years of specialising, that the largest group of women with eating disorders are those who are not generally recognised as sick, i.e. not the obese nor the anorexic, but the women of average weight whose obsession with remaining 'normal' takes over their lives . . . the successful dieters . . . the women who insist that they are fat when they are clearly not, who talk about their 'gross thighs' or stomach or

hips . . . whose remarks in the presence of food are . . . always predictable: 'Think of the calories in this'; 'Oh no, I never eat pudding, I have to watch my figure.'

Women are extraordinarily good at hiding these things. Three perfectly ordinary, attractive women involved in the production of this book each wrote secretly offering their own sad tales. Sometimes they would even be funny if they weren't so serious. Rosalind has a typically unbalanced attitude to food, even though she is very slim. One day she was given a large box of chocolates. This posed a dilemma: she adored chocolates but didn't want to put on weight. So, after hours of agonizing, she decided she'd be *very* strong and indulge in the luxury of one chocolate a day. This went well for four days until she had to go out for the evening, and returned with happy expectations of a chocolate.

'Chocolates?' said her husband casually from behind his newspaper. 'Oh, I finished them.' And then to compound this felony, he added, 'You shouldn't be eating them anyway.'

Maddened to a frenzy, Rosalind actually took up a kitchen knife and went for him. No damage was done, and the story would seem incomprehensible to anybody who has a balanced attitude to food. But I've told this dreadful, lovely tale to a dozen women, and most – laughing heartily as well – understand it perfectly.

With stories like these cropping up by the score, my own straightforward history of yo-yo dieting paled into insignificance. What a tragic waste of time and happiness! I am not claiming that women with disordered eating are constantly unhappy, though some certainly are. What I am saying is that even my own concerns with dieting significantly interfered with an otherwise happy life. After all, there are aspects of one's life it's possible to forget sometimes, but never one's body: it's always there, for all to see.

In Princess Diana's case, her eating disorder appears to have been brought on, in part, by the pressures of her job and marriage, but it often happens the other way round. Peter Grose-Hodge, past-president of the International Academy of Matrimonial Lawyers, remarked in the *Guardian* on the increasingly familiar type of woman who, having been 'slightly anorexic – like so many stylish women who semi-starve themselves', goes on to become bulimic in her forties, with the result that her marriage breaks up. Other examples of disordered eaters are the housewives who, busy feeding the family, are rarely seen to sit down and eat themselves.

They disguise their eating disorders with comments such as 'You go on, I had my food in the kitchen while I was cooking'. Or there is the young woman at a dinner party who claims to have such a weak bladder that she must rush to the loo after each course. Perhaps she is telling the truth, but it is odd that she is gone so long, and that she returns to the table looking slightly flushed. Yesterday I dined at a restaurant only to find that the ladies' loo was blocked with vomit; twice recently I have heard the sounds of retching from the next-door loo. Yes, it may have been the lousy food, and I am certainly not trying to be alarmist. Perhaps my real message is that so much of women's odd eating behaviour has been going on so long that we have ceased to regard it as abnormal (only a paragraph back I referred to my yo-yo dieting as comparatively 'insignificant'). After all, women habitually put up with discomforts that men would never countenance. But we *must* recognize disordered eating for what it is: at best, a serious impediment to enjoying life and, at worst, lethal.

Anorexia burgeoned as a middle-class condition in the Twenties and Thirties, shrank back during the war, then returned in the Sixties, and is now spreading all around the social spectrum and across the sexes. Although 95 per cent of adult sufferers are women the proportion of younger males is higher: 10 per cent of teenagers and a full 25 per cent of pre-teen anorexics are boys. That's a very dramatic rise. There is strong evidence that as the obsession with slenderness continues, adult men are dieting as never before, though secretly.

Because anorexia and bulimia are seen as 'self-inflicted' they do not arouse anything like the sympathy that other conditions can expect. But they are not self-inflicted. They are inflicted by fashion: every year, every month, every week, every day, every hour, every minute, the constant, unremitting, crushing pressure to be thin and glamorous takes its toll. The rights and wrongs of cigarette smoking are hotly debated – after all, opponents argue, smoking threatens the health and lives of our children. Yet anorexia destroys bodies *and* minds, not over a lifetime, but very, very quickly. In 1990, the American Anorexia and Bulimia Association calculated that some degree of anorexia or bulimia strikes a million American women every year; 30,000 also become emetic abusers. Every year 150,000 American women die of anorexia. That's about 0.05 per cent of the population. Even the most conservative estimates calculate that at least 1 per cent of women have anorexia, of which as many as one-fifth will die. As Naomi Wolf points out, according to the Anorexia and Bulimia Association, that means in America there were 17,024 *more* anorexic deaths than the total number of deaths from AIDS tabulated by the World Health Organisation in 177 countries and territories from the beginning of the epidemic until the end of 1988.

Once you are on the lookout, statistics overwhelm you. I have, in fact, omitted many of those I collected, lest readers suspect me of being in the grip of a loony conspiracy theory. But they are all well-attested, mostly medical, statistics. Some commentators believe that up to 10 per cent of all American females are anorexic to some degree, and that on university campuses the figure goes up to 20 per cent. Anorexia strikes hardest at the intelligent, high achievers of the middle classes. There are even more bulimics: up to 20 per cent of American college women binge and purge on a regular basis. In *The Hungry Self*, Kim Chernin suggests that at least half the women on campuses in the United States suffer at some time from bulimia or anorexia. After yet more statistics Naomi Wolf concludes that

> it means that of ten young American women in college, two will be anorexic and six will be bulimic; only two will be well. The norm, then, for young, middle-class American women, is to be a sufferer from some form of eating disease.

Around half the number of anorexics never recover completely; once anorexic, their lives are permanently blighted by an obsession from which they cannot free themselves, their bodies damaged beyond repair. The symptoms are most unpleasant, including loss of periods, hyperactivity, abdominal pain and swelling, insomnia, constipation, dizzy spells, growth of fine downy hair on the body and loss of hair on the head, poor circulation, rough pale skin, severe mood swings. Long-term effects include osteoporosis, sterility, severe depression, even gangrene and, of course, death.

But that's America and they do things differently there. We are very much better off. We have only 3.5 million anorexics or bulimics, a mere 6000 new cases yearly. Around 40 per cent will recover after an average illness of five years, but up to 20 per cent will die: half from suicide. And not only are numbers rising each year, but patients are now *thinner* than ever before. In this century, America has always led in matters of weight, but Britain follows close

behind. These are not odd people, nutcases or adolescent neur-
otics. Sufferers aged from six to eighty have been reported. They
tend to be conscientious and well-behaved high achievers and to
come from close-knit families. Back in the Seventies three of my
schoolfriends had to be taken away because, as I later learned, they
had become anorexic. All three were (and this is not sentimental
nostalgia, but hard fact) among the cleverest, best-looking, most
talented, humorous, *slimmest* girls in the class.

I don't know where these three girls are now, or if they are alive.

It is not only Britain and America. The number of women
sufferers has increased dramatically throughout the industrial
world: Russia, Australia, Sweden, Italy all have harrowing statistics,
especially among teenagers. Dramatic though the numbers are,
the most alarming aspect is the speed of the increase. The Netherlands has seen a rise of 400 per cent in ten years. I mentioned
earlier the plight of young Japanese girls, starving their curves
away in spite of the pleas of their parents, teachers and boyfriends.
Most Western women diet at some time in their lives, the vast
majority unnecessarily and virtually all without success. 'The
number of eating-disordered patients in a given community,' writes
Professor Hsu of the University of Pittsburgh School of Medicine,
'occurs in proportion to the number of individuals who are
dieting.'

How tragic that at the very time when women are making their
mark as never before, in surveys they repeatedly insist that they
value losing weight above success in love and above success in
work. This is bimbo-think. I can't help recalling those brave suffra-
gettes who, at the turn of the century, endured the agonies of
hunger strikes and force-feeding in order that women should have
equal opportunities. How ironic that this is what we have come to.

A Magic Way to Lose Weight?

'Princess Diana does it and what a beautiful figure she has! She
may have been driven to bulimia by an unhappy marriage, but as
a slimming device being sick obviously works!'

I've heard this comment many times recently. A decade ago
'anorexia' was the 'in' word. Now, in the last few years, 'bulimia'
has shot ahead, cropping up constantly in magazines and TV
programmes. Full-blown bulimia is three times more common

than anorexia, although these days more and more bulimics are going on to develop anorexia. Induced vomiting and laxative abuse are on the increase. Some women binge ten or more times a day, shovelling in up to 32,000 calories a day.

Bulimia not only has horrendous side effects, it's a lousy way to get thin. I know a thing or two about the subject, because for many years, long before Lady Diana had even met Prince Charles, I was convinced I'd discovered a miraculous way to lose weight. The result? I gained weight, *and* started losing control of my eating.

My near entry into bulimia was, I imagine, not a common route, but it illustrates how very simple it is to get there. It began with travel sickness. When I was a child, ten minutes in a motorcar, five minutes on the bus or two minutes in a taxi rendered me very ill indeed. My childhood memories of school outings consist of a pleasant setting off, chatting and laughing with my friends, then a gradual, horrible onset of sickness. Bit by bit it crept up on me while I sat in misery trying desperately to avoid looking at the scores of greasy sausage advertisements flashing past. After a very long period of slow, miserable torture, often as much as half an hour or forty-five minutes (a lifetime for a nine-year-old) the nausea got so bad that eventually, *eventually*, I had to stop the car, get out, and stand ignominiously beside the road waiting. If I was very lucky I might actually *be* sick. *Being* sick provides almost instant relief from *feeling* sick. You can then crawl back into the car, shaking and weak but definitely a lot better. There are five or ten minutes of a pleasant journey before the whole ghastly process begins again. So, though most people regard vomiting as a beastly business, early on I learned to associate being sick with feeling better, a feeling of absolute relief, of freedom and lightness.

When I was older it was a small step from there to using induced vomiting in other situations. I call them Christmas Day occasions: days when, having stuffed oneself on turkey and pudding, one is fit for nothing more lively than slumping in front of the television. Not me – I'd nip off to the bathroom, do my bit, and come back beaming with good health. Come teatime, I was as hungry as an ox and could enjoy my food all over again, while everyone else was feeling like a foie gras goose.

There's a distinguished historical precedent for this. Two thousand years ago the Romans, having gorged themselves, would saunter off to the vomitorium to be sick before starting to stuff all over again. Even before then, ancient Egyptian papyruses suggest several means of emptying the stomach – infusion of fennel and honey, crude sea salt, and other such – not in order to prolong the pleasure of eating but for medicinal purposes. For centuries, vomiting has been prescribed by doctors as a means of curing disease, or for simply maintaining good health; indeed for most of medical history the two mainstays of medicine were vomiting and purging. The seventeenth-century French dramatist Molière wrapped up all therapy of his time in a Latin formula which loosely translates to mean 'enema, then bleed, and finally purge'.

In some cultures vomiting is still encouraged. Some years ago an academic friend of mine paid a visit to a remote part of China. A large and impressive banquet was laid out for him. One course followed on another until he felt he could eat no more. Then a large tureen was placed in the centre of the table. A servant lifted the lid, and lo and behold twenty tiny baby mice scampered out. My friend turned pale: he'd heard unpleasant stories about the variety of animals that the Chinese like to eat. But good manners were paramount and he copied his hosts as they leaned across, lifted a baby mouse by the tail, opened their mouths and lowered the mice down their throats. Only in the nick of time did my friend realize that the rodents were not for consumption, but, with their wiggling whiskers and legs, to induce vomiting.

Nowadays most women use their fingers. (Bite marks around the knuckles are often the first signs another person notices.) Over 1000 years ago, Avicenna, in his Canon of Medicine, recommended using a feather if one ate to excess, but even he recognized it to be dangerous if done more than once or twice a month, not only because it quickly becomes addictive but because it is 'injurious to the stomach . . . and may lead to consumption. The custom of some people who eat to excess and then procure vomiting is one of the things that end in a chronic disorder'.

There are many complaints associated with bulimia: ruined teeth from the acid in the vomit (dentists are often the first health professionals to notice signs of bulimia), swollen glands, low blood potassium levels which can disturb the heart's rhythm and even lead to sudden death, swollen, infected salivary glands, bleeding and tears in the oesophagus, and stomach ulcers, to name but a few. One young sufferer, quoted in *Woman's Own* last year, admitted:

> Physically, I doubt my body will ever recover – I have chronic bowel problems, my teeth are capped where stomach

acid from being sick wore the enamel away and my bone density is low for my age . . .

Doctors have recently seen a terrible new trend, as described by Professor Hubert Lacy of St George's Hospital in London:

> The number of bulimics damaging themselves by self-muti-lation, drink and drugs has more than trebled over the past seven years . . . I believe women are expected to achieve academically, at work, and in sexual and maternal matters without the usual assertiveness shown by men. Some patients seem to turn that assertiveness on themselves.

Many women are aware of the terrible effects of bulimia, but the lure of a skinny figure plus the ability to eat as much as they want is enough justification and to hell with the consequences. As one woman put it:

> They say it ruins your teeth, but Princess Di has a lovely set of teeth and quite frankly why should I worry about some mythical future problems when I'm miserable now because I feel I'm too fat. Diana's done it and she looks great. That's good enough for me.

Another pointed out to me:

> I was sick every day of my pregnancy. Don't tell me that being sick can be that bad for you.

It *is* that bad for you. By the time those nasty side effects have struck and you're wishing you'd never started, it's too late. Quite apart from those, nine times out of ten *vomiting doesn't work as a slimming method.* Calories are absorbed very fast indeed: up to 20 or 30 per cent of the energy of what you eat can be taken in before you even get to the lavatory.

You may decide, as I did (being sensible), to restrict your vomiting to one meal a day. After all, I reasoned, it's only the same as missing a meal and that's not harmful. But I can virtually guarantee that you will not stop there. You begin by sicking up a meal sometimes: a very big one, or a very calorific one, the one where you happen to have eaten all that ice cream. After a while you're tempted to do it more and more. Writes Mrs Wheeler, of Sheffield:

> You eat a lovely, big meal, then you get rid of it. Incidentally the more you eat the easier it is to sick it up, so it encourages you to really scoff. You may be happy with this for a week or two. You don't feel hungry immediately afterwards. That's the beauty of it. But you do an hour or two later. Very hungry. Why not eat again? That demon in your brain will start whispering in your ear – 'You've only had fifty calories today. Why not just eat another meal and do the same?' You very quickly get into a vicious circle of stuffing and vomiting.

Mrs Hanson from Cardiff summed up:

> At the most basic level you don't lose weight, because your body *does* absorb some calories from all those meals. Plus you're spending three times the amount on food. Plus you have a filthy lavatory to clean every day. Plus you are boosting your obsession with eating, sending it rocketing sky-high, when what you need to be doing is getting away from obsessions with food.

Incredible though it sounds, it is not unknown for women to turn to crime to support their eating obsessions. One recent confession in a popular magazine described how the compulsive eater, when she ran out of money, took to eating scraps of food she found in the street, and then turned to prostitution to feed her habit. 'For a treat I'd chill a block of butter and eat it in slices,' she recalled.

For me, the turning point from convenience to addiction came when I felt tarnished if I didn't make myself sick. It was a creeping, sticky, clinging sort of feeling. Claustrophobic. Contaminated. I couldn't think of anything else with that food sitting there inside me. I couldn't relax. It began to rule my day. When I started I thought I'd do it every other day. This quickly progressed to the stage that if I ate a meal, a meal that I badly needed, not simply for nutritional reasons (desperate dieters don't give a damn about those) but to stop my body going into starvation mode and putting on weight, then I felt fat, cloyish and oppressed if the food remained inside me. So I would have the choice: either get rid of it and end up eating very little, or spend the rest of the day feeling contaminated and obsessed.

This change in psychology can happen very, very quickly. I was lucky – or strong-willed – and simply forced myself to stop. I never got into the secret binges and purges, the massive meals consumed and then emitted. I never felt the terrible self-disgust that some women feel. But many times I pulled myself from the brink of such behaviour just in time. It is a very, very frightening feeling.

So don't get into the habit of making yourself sick or taking laxatives. It won't make you thin and it's every bit as dangerous as drug abuse. Treat your body with more respect and dignity.

12
Our Children's Health

Y ou may yourself be one of the few non-dieting women. Or, if you do diet, you may feel that this is your choice, and that you do not object to the constant pressure to be super-thin, though (if so) I'm not sure why you are reading this book.

What nobody has a right to do is to inflict their obsession on the next generation.

Karen is thirty-four years old. She grew up in a family that considered skinniness essential for a woman:

> For years in my teens and twenties I dieted and criticized my body. My mother had always been concerned about her glamorous image and I took this as the normal way to be. But in the last few years I've realized what a debilitating pressure this has been. I've wasted years of my life caught up in it when I could have been happy and self-confident. I know it sounds awful, but I hate my mother for it, even though she was herself a victim. I blame her, and when I see other parents foisting these values on their children, it breaks my heart.

The effects on our children of dieting begin before they are born. Today's obsession with unnatural slenderness is not simply a matter of vanity, or even of our own health. It is an issue which concerns the mental and physical health of all successive generations. The scientific literature on the subject is growing rapidly. What follows is merely a sampling of some of the more remarkable facts about dieting, children and adolescents that have recently been coming to light. I'll start at the very beginning of the process with . . .

Sexual Desire: 'Studies consistently show that with dietary deprivation, sexual interests dissipate.' One study revealed that women often stopped masturbating or having sexual fantasies below 1700 calories a day.

Conception: Dieting can have dramatic effects on female fertility. One of the ways in which the body makes metabolic adjustments to counteract the effects of dieting is by disrupting the menstrual cycle, and infertility is unusually common even in 'ideal' weight women who are chronic dieters. Weight gain will often result in conception in such cases, though, because so many doctors have unthinkingly joined the slenderness bandwagon, it is rarely recommended. Menopause also comes earlier in thinner women and women who have lost weight by dieting.

In Chapter 5 I revealed that an infertility study had shown that out of twenty-nine previously infertile women, twenty-six conceived on giving up their dieting and gaining a few pounds.

Pregnancy: Diets are particularly dangerous during pregnancy, when women need the extra calories because of the energy required to produce a baby. Low-carbohydrate diets are especially dangerous, since the biological effect of carbohydrate deprivation (ketosis) can damage the foetus. One of the most exciting areas of medical research concerns the astonishing discovery that what you eat when you are pregnant can affect the health of your *grandchildren*.

Birth: Just as fertility appears to be greatest in plump women, so does the chance of a successful pregnancy. Obstetric complications are much more common among the lean, and underweight women double their risk of low-birth-weight babies.

One to five years: Nowadays children as young as *two* have already begun to adopt a dislike of fatness which they have learned from adults. This is unfortunate because children tend naturally to prefer the comfort of a large person. But 'parents are afraid and ashamed of heavy children', writes the psychologist Susan Wooley, who spent three days in public places such as a zoo and amusement park asking parents for permission to photograph their child. 'No parent of a lean child ever refused; no parent of an overweight child ever agreed.' The first pre-schooler's book on slimming was

214

published in 1972 by Mary Lynn Solot, called *100 Hamburgers: The Getting Thin Book*, though most overweight infants become normal-weight children.

The pressure on girls to eat less than is normal, and less well than they should, begins very early. Looking at a sample of babies in America, it was found that 99 per cent of the boys were breast-fed, but only 66 per cent of the girls, and, further, that the girls were given half the time to feed.

Seven years: By the age of seven adult perceptions of attractiveness are accepted. In an investigation of school children by Michael Maloney, of the Children's Hospital Medical Center in Cincinnati, 41 per cent of the girls between seven and twelve had dieted, the *average age* at which they started being nine years and seven months. Anybody over thirty years old who casts their mind back to what they were doing at seven, eight or nine years old will appreciate just how terrible this is. Cases of anorexics as young as seven and a half have been reported. The age of first-time dieters has decreased rapidly in the last decade (when I was at school in the late Sixties most dieters didn't begin until fifteen or sixteen), and the dramatic increase of pre-puberty dieting is particularly alarming from the point of view of mental and physical health.

Eight years: The author of *The Beverly Hills Diet* began dieting when she was eight. By the time she left high school she was 'on everything: thyroid pills, diet pills, laxatives'. Known also as the anorexics diet and the diarrhoea diet, this book sold millions in America despite wide condemnation in the medical press.

Nine years: The desire for thinness is starting to set in with most girls, as well as concerns about dieting. It now has less to do with weight, and more with fashion. Hips are disliked. Half of the girls who want to slim are normal weight. Even underweight girls may begin toying with diets. Often these diets are broken by episodes of bingeing. 'At best we are conferring on some a lifetime of dispute and discontent with their physical appearance and eating behaviour,' writes Andrew Hill in the *British Journal of Clinical Psychology*. 'At worst, there is the potential for an explosion in clinical eating problems and disorders.' In another article, he notes that of a sample of nearly 400 nine-year-old children, the girls already wanted to weigh 11 per cent less than the average for

215

their age. Psychiatrists Achenbach and Howell have shown that major depressions in later life can often be traced back to low self-esteem beginning at about nine years old.

Recently, there have been several reports of women committing suicide because they consider themselves too ugly to live. These women tend to be young and pretty. But mere prettiness has made them dangerously self-critical. Instead of accepting their looks and getting on with life, they begin to think obsessively that if only they could change this or that, then they would be beautiful. It doesn't work. They break up.

Ten years: When I was in my late teens and living at home there used to be a little girl, about ten years old, who lived nearby. Evidently her parents were something in the way of slave drivers, for we used frequently to see her lugging heavy bags of shopping about. Once, to our great surprise, while we were walking the dogs at close on midnight, we saw her coming home alone, quite fancily dressed in evening clothes and carrying a little handbag.

Years passed: the little girl showed no signs of growing. It was only then that we discovered that she was in fact the same age as I was, but that at a very young age she had suffered severe anorexia. This had so disrupted her growth and hormones that she remained looking like an undeveloped ten-year-old.

Some girls are beginning to see themselves as fatter than they are (this is known as body-size overestimation). In a well-known experiment conducted in the Sixties, and since replicated, ten- and eleven-year-old children were asked to rank in order of approval six line drawings of children – one average, four handicapped, and one overweight. The overweight child was consistently ranked last, below the child in leg brace and crutches, or in a wheelchair, or missing a hand, or with facial disfigurement.

The National Association of Anorexia Nervosa and Associated Disorders reports that 'preadolescent dieting has increased "exponentially" in recent years'.

A survey of 494 middle-class school girls in San Francisco found that more than half described themselves as overweight, while only 15 per cent were by medical standards; 81 per cent of ten-year-olds were dieters.

Eleven years: Of the London schoolgirls aged between eleven and eighteen interviewed by psychiatrist Andrew Hill, 59 per cent said they wanted to lose weight, and over half of the average-weight girls said that they felt fat. The average age at which anorexia begins for children treated at Great Ormond Street Hospital is eleven. By the time they get to the hospital 90 per cent are emaciated. It is estimated that anorexia affects 20,000 British school children. While 10 per cent of teenage anorexics are boys, the figure goes up to 25 per cent among pre-teen boys, thus showing an alarming trend.

Puberty: With puberty, the period of greatest danger begins. The fact that hormonal changes result in almost a trebling of the amount of her body fat at the very time when girls are particularly aware of their appearance leads to a strong motivation to diet. But dieting during this vital period of hormonal change can damage the body permanently.

Parents are not always helpful. Fathers make remarks about chubbiness, which, even in jest, can cause a child considerable distress and lead to self-disgust. The children of chronic-dieting mothers tend to become chronic dieters themselves. Some parents want their children to look like models as soon as they show signs of ending childhood, if not before. You see it frequently in the celebrity magazines such as *Hello!*. As part of their image and for good publicity, socialites and stars often make their little girls dress up like a miniature sex-pusses, already dieting and revealing bits of pubescent skin. I've had many letters from women who remember one or other (or both) of their parents starting, very early on, to make snide remarks and taunts about the daughter's weight, encouraging her to go on a diet even if she was only slightly plump (which it is very healthy for a young girl to be). It's rarely done with the son, but often with the daughter.

A new disorder is appearing in the chapters on anorexia and bulimia in the medical textbooks: baryophobia, or the fear of becoming heavy. The children who suffer from baryophobia are stunted in growth and sexual development (thus potentially affecting the third generation). They are undernourished, either due to their own fear of becoming fat or because their parents fear they will grow fat or develop heart disease and a high cholesterol level. Two paediatricians, Deitz and Hartnung, at Tufts University School of Medicine, Boston, discovered '*that even mildly restrictive diets may be associated with a reduction in linear growth velocity*', while they note that 'highly restrictive diets in younger children have

217

almost uniformly been associated with marked decreases in height velocity'.

Parents will sometimes encourage or allow their children to follow the same slimming or healthy, low-fat diets that adults use without realizing that the calorie requirements for a growing child are greater and much more critical than they are for an adult. Dr Dee Dawson, who runs Rhodes Farm, an eating-disorder unit for children, says, 'Kids are picking up on the healthy eating messages aimed at adults and cutting out fat and sugar. I've had girls here who've lost half their body weight – from 8 st to 4 st – but still don't realize the harm they're doing.'

Not only does dieting mess around with the metabolism and central nervous system of the growing child, possibly resulting in eating disorders and diminished growth, but there is also now a suggestion, reported in the American specialist journal *Pediatrics*, 'that failure to gain weight normally during puberty, per se, predisposes the patient to reduced skeletal mass and an increased risk of osteoporosis later in life.'

The fact is that no one knows what is the best weight for the average child at a given age, or even whether the idea is meaningful. All the weight tables for children and adolescents are guesswork. This is in part because evidence is extremely difficult to collect, but largely because during the first two decades, more than at any other time, individuals vary enormously in their physical requirements.

Twelve years: By this age girls are often dieting to the same degree as adult women, and in the hopes of reaching an abnormally low weight. (Boys are more concerned about their height.) They are also starting to feel guilty about eating. Very recently, a study carried out by Alison Field, of Harvard University, revealed that up to two-thirds of *underweight* girls between ten and twelve considered themselves too heavy.

Thirteen years: About half of girls, irrespective of their actual weight, are unhappy with their bodies. Soon this will become normal for girls – i.e. most will feel dissatisfied with their size. Half of normal-weight girls want to lose more than one-tenth of their body weight. Adolescent girls in Western societies, as well as in increasingly Westernized Japan, are, in general, unhappier and much more self-critical than boys.

218

Fourteen years: By now focused dissatisfactions have intensified, particularly with regard to hips and thighs. Fifty per cent of adolescent girls have started dieting before the age of fifteen, despite the fact that it can be very bad for their health and growth. About a fifth of these will turn into adolescent chronic dieters, who are nearly ten times more likely to use vomiting and laxative abuse as slimming methods.

Fifteen years: The relative risk of dieters at this age becoming anorexics and bulimics is eight times that of non-dieters. As many as 80 per cent of normal-weight and 40 per cent of underweight fifteen-year-olds have dieted to lose weight. What matters is not actual body weight so much as perceived body weight. Feeling fat even when you're not has now become common.

Sixteen years: In California, 10 per cent of high-school girls vomit and 7 per cent abuse laxatives in order to lose weight. However, in common with adults, many pre-adolescent and adolescent dieters do not eat less than non-dieters, only much more erratically. The combination of living in a world where delicious food is everywhere and attempting not to eat when you're hungry is too difficult to maintain.

Seventeen years: By late adolescence only three out of ten girls have not been on a diet. Up to eight out of ten feel themselves too fat, compared with only a quarter of the boys. Write Drs Casper and Offer in *Pediatrics*: 'Overall, the findings suggest that preoccupation with weight and/or dieting concerns in either male or female adolescents is likely to indicate psychological problems.'

Eighteen years and over: The minority of women questioned at universities and colleges have normal eating habits, with up to a quarter displaying mild symptoms of bulimic behaviour, though only about 5 per cent have fully fledged bulimia. Bingeing, vomiting, chronic dieting and laxative abuse are all fairly common. Not only are they common, they are rapidly increasing. In a survey of 33,000 American women, only 7.6 per cent over thirty years old reported vomiting for weight control. Nearly 20 per cent under the age of twenty had done so. Perceptions of weight are also becoming more seriously askew. One American study found that although college women were on average 5 per cent *below* their recommended weights, 85 per cent considered themselves to be slightly or seriously overweight. In a British study, it was found that up to 90 per cent of women want to weigh less than the average and are, in their slimming concerns, inseparable from bulimics. Eighteen is also the average age for onset of anorexia, which in teenagers is ten and a half times more common in girls. Nineteen is the average age of onset for bulimia, from which about 5 per cent of the adult female population suffer.

Girls of university age have, according to research,

> only one overriding concern: the shape and weight of their bodies. They all wanted to lose 5–25 pounds, even though most [were] not remotely overweight. They went into great detail about every flaw in their anatomies, and told of the great disgust they felt every time they looked in the mirror.
>
> *Face Value: The Politics of Beauty*

At eighteen-plus women are starting to have children of their own – and so the cycle begins all over again . . .

We Are All Involved!

It is not only parents that are concerned in this. Unless we all – mothers, fathers, grandparents, aunts and uncles, cousins, brothers, sisters, schoolteachers, youth leaders – call a halt to the insanity of excess dieting, unless we insist that the pressure being brought to bear on young people to be unrealistically thin is stopped, then we must hold ourselves responsible for psychologically and physically maiming, in some cases even killing, our children, our coming generation.

Part Three

WHAT REALLY WORKS?

13

Start Today!

Diets don't work. They make you obsessed with food; they upset the chemical balance and regulatory mechanisms of your body; they are antisocial, unpleasant, ineffective, sometimes dangerous, always difficult, and quite often make you fatter than you were to begin with. Buy a slimming book with 'diet' in the title, and you waste your money as well as your peace of mind.

I hope that this book has shown that the current fashion for super-skinniness is neither healthy nor admirable. But what to do if you still feel, in spite of it all, that you need to lose weight?

That's where my plan comes in.

Remember what I said in the Diet Digest about packaging diets? So often they exclaim that they're revolutionary, and have scientific mumbo-jumbo and dazzling statistics to back them up, as well as a mountain of testimonials. Well, before I give you the details about my plan, let me subject it to a Diet-Digest analysis.

First, this is a balanced, non-calorie-counting, no-set-menus plan which concentrates on painlessly ensuring that your food is tasty, plentiful, healthy and the most likely to help you lose excess weight for good. It is also an exercise plan. But once again it's not about the production of a starry-eyed, emaciated zealot. Believe me, I know only too well how hard it is to change habits. That's why this plan is relaxed, very simple to follow (hence, why this part of the book is so short) and will not interfere with your life in the way that ordinary diets do. It is really more a sensible set of guidelines than anything else.

It is not revolutionary. It is perfectly straightforward, and without gimmicks.

Further, this plan will not turn you into a supermodel by the end of the week. But then, as you know very well, neither will the latest diet book no matter what superlatives the cover blurb uses. What this plan will do is help you, over a twelve-week period, to break out of the dieting and guzzling habit, and get back in control of food. If you're supermodel material, then that is your best chance of losing weight without losing your looks too.

The Importance of Language

Studies have shown that men have a far more positive self-image than women. When a group of people are asked to comment on their physical attractiveness, the men tend to describe their good points, which are usually (in their own eyes) quite numerous: 'I have nice hair, good shoulders, well-shaped hands', and so on. Women, on the other hand – even the most attractive women – almost unanimously describe themselves very critically in terms of their 'defects': 'My bum's too big, I have cellulite, my hair's too thin', and so forth.

Needless to say, these subjective descriptions often bear little relation to what the person looks like to others. I've often been amazed at the self-confidence and high opinion of themselves that some ugly, greasy-haired old men seem to have! Well, we women need to cultivate a bit of that too.

Now here is an exercise: go and look at yourself in the mirror and start enumerating your good features. If necessary, get together with a friend who can help point out what may be invisible to you. I can virtually guarantee that you are your severest critic, and that other people see you far more positively than you do. Now *remember* those good points at all times. As for your less pleasing features, it is far better simply to ignore them. Books and articles that dwell on endless subterfuges and disguises ('Ten Top Tips for Tiny Tits' I once read) are counterproductive because they make you obsessed with your so-called 'defects'. Take a flattering photo of yourself, dressed and made up in the way that suits you best. If you've got a bit of spare cash, get your photograph taken professionally, soft-focus lights, romantic mistiness, painted backdrop and all, if you like. When you've a set of snaps you like, leave them around. Just concentrate on what you like about yourself and reserve your mental energies for better things than worrying about what you cannot change.

Once you've had enough of that, start thinking about how you would describe yourself. Not just your hair, leg length and so forth, but your *overall* description. I want to dwell on this, because the *words* we use to describe our own and other people's bodies are extremely important. Language not only reflects how we think, it conditions and forms our minds. Yet in the past few decades the language we use to describe ourselves has narrowed miserably. Women nowadays are

> *thin*
> or
> *fat*

These are the 'real' words of today. Pauline, in company, described herself as 'statuesque' and was sharply rebuked for being euphemistic. 'What you mean is you're big – no, let's not beat about the bush: fat. You need to lose weight.' Pauline is not fat. She does not need to lose weight, and the dreary word 'big' tells us nothing. Statuesque describes her perfectly.

In the past, physical descriptions of people were far more sensitive to the person as a whole, noting a man or woman's expression, their carriage, how they moved, details of their complexion, the intelligence in their eyes – all the variety of details that make an *individual.* Witness this description of Queen Elizabeth I:

> Shee was a lady, upon whom nature had bestowed, and well placed, many of her fayrest favores; of stature meane, slender, streight, and amiably composed; of such state in her carriage, as every motione of her seemed to beare majesty: her Haire was inclined to pale yellow, her forehead large and faire, a seemeing sete for princely grace; her eyes lively and sweete, but short-sighted; her nose somewhat rising in the middest; the whole compasse of her countenance somewhat long, but yet of an admirable beauty, not so much in that which is tearmed the flower of youth, as in a most delightfull compositione of majesty and modesty in equall mixture.
>
> Sir John Hayward

Such descriptions are a delight to read, not least because they suggest appreciation above censure. Of course, I'm not suggesting that we all go around speaking in ye olde English – 'Gad zooks!'

and 'Fie, Sir Charles' – simply that we might try to regain some of the old subtlety of description. What makes people acceptable today, alas, is their uniformity.

So, let's begin by abandoning those bland, narrow little designations 'thin' and 'fat' and start to use words that actually tell us something about the individual, words that can also conjure colours and textures, the whole person, clothes, style and all. I consulted a thesaurus and found instead of fat:

Statuesque	Curvaceous	Radiant	Comely
Shapely	Well-favoured	Stately	Majestic
Ornamental	Exquisite	Resplendent	Dazzling
Gorgeous	Buxom	Classical	Magnificent
Splendid	Large	Voluptuous	Handsome
Aphrodite	Amazonian	Substantial	Delectable
Strapping	Robust	Tigress	Rounded

In describing yourself I am not suggesting that you kid yourself. You may feel that you are unequivocally stout/podgy/hefty/plump, but that you are *also* voluptuous. Or, more likely, you may say, yes, indeed my legs are on the stocky side and would benefit from a quick *Tour de France*, but overall I am simply *magnificent*. If no word quite fits you, make one up. A large woman I know unblushingly refers to herself as 'quilted'.

The words above are more often associated with plenty and fullness in women, but there are elegant words to describe skinnies:

Fiddlestring	Sinewy	Serpentine	Svelte
Slinky	Willowy	Rangy	Lean

My favourite description of a skinny person is 'she has to run round in the shower to get wet'.

For those of you who are on the large size, let me remind you that there are plenty of critical words for skinnies:

Scrawny	Beanpole	Scraggy	Broomhandle
Emaciated	Scarecrow	Rake	Shadow
Wraith	Haggard	Lanky	Bony
Weedy	Pinched	Cadaverous	Raw-boned
Wizened	Withered	Peaky	Pencil

Wasted   Skeleton   Deflated   Stick

In short, it's not the state of thinness or fatness that's important, it's how you describe it.

These new words need not apply only to yourself but also to your friends, because the more we create an atmosphere of tolerance, the more we ourselves benefit. This is an area where we are lucky today. Rita, who grew up after the war, comments:

> In the Fifties, when there was a big drive to re-domesticate women, there was so much more backbiting, perhaps as a result of women being discouraged from having jobs, or any interests outside sewing and cooking. Men were regarded as objects of the chase, and other women as rivals and enemies. We were constantly making snide comments about each other such as 'Mutton dressed as lamb' and so on. The result was, you lived in an atmosphere in which you felt you too were constantly being criticized and undermined.

The more we accept other women's figures – however odd or unfashionable – the closer we are to beating this ludicrous drive for one uniform, skeletal figure, that oppresses us all. Telling other people they ought to diet is playing into the hands of the dieting industry. Living as I do in a university town, I am struck by the fact that among the scores of young women who worry themselves sick about their figures, there is a bold, brave, *intelligent* minority who are saying, 'What the hell. I'm going to dress comfortably, eat what I like and still be beautiful.'

Each one of us who has the courage to say *enough is enough* is making a gesture for *all* women. One less gaunt woman on the streets will help to turn the tide. One anti-dieting gesture at a dinner party may influence another woman away from a needless diet. Take my hairdresser Lidia for example. She's voluptuous, happy and healthy. When busybody strangers start telling her to diet she suppresses her irritation at their intrusion and replies reasonably: 'I don't need to diet.' Often, this sets them thinking, questioning why indeed if we are happy and healthy we must starve and be miserable. We need more Lidias to speak out.

Collect Pictures of Beautiful Non-Skinnies

You'd be surprised how much this simple, rather juvenile trick can do for your confidence. I already mentioned in Chapter 3 how encouraging it is to read magazines like *Yes!*, which specialize in clothes for and articles about size 16+ women. Even if you're a size 8, it's very liberating to realize that women of even size 20+ can look gorgeous. And I don't mean gorgeous in the patronizing way, either. I mean seriously beautiful, just as today's models are seriously beautiful. The first issue I bought had pictures of a fashion show. There, in bold colour, full frontal, dressed in tight-fitting leggings, was an extremely beautiful model who must have been at least a size 18. It did wonders for my self-confidence. She was buxom, certainly, and had very big thighs, without a doubt; but she would have had any one of the men I know at her beck and call if she'd come through my front door. It came as little surprise to me when I later discovered that one of the blokes I'd shown the photo to had later stolen the whole magazine!

Also try writing to shops which sell size 16+ clothes to get a copy of their catalogue. If they also sell smaller sizes, then the chances are that they'll only use smaller-sizes in the catalogue, but if they specialize in size 16+, then their catalogue is likely to be filled with lots of inspiring figures. Look at them whenever you're feeling low. It will restore your mood and stop you from getting into an obsession with dieting and, hence, an obsession with food.

Try pornography magazines, if you don't mind reaching up that high in the newsagent's. Certainly, these contain lots of sprawling skinnies exposing all their bits, but there are also plenty of bigger women, looking just as enticing.

Back to more respectable areas, just think of the opera singer Jessye Norman. Look through the art section in the bookshop or library. Lord Clarke's book *The Nude* – an eminently respectable study of how, since earliest civilized times, art has depicted the human body – has piles of pictures of big beauties, little beauties, in-between beauties, just to confirm once again that you don't have to be a blonde size 10, to have good facial structure and an enticing body.

Wear the Clothes You Want to Wear

There's no doubt that the clothes we choose to wear are often symbolic of our mood. They reflect our self-regard, our inhibitions (or lack of them), our joys, disappointments, and, above all, our confidence. The shapeless, drab horrors so many women go in for when they're feeling fat serve only to make them feel worse: more frumpy, more hopeless, more prone to comfort eating. The more you equate your true size with a sense of failure and cowering, the worse you make your life and the lives of other 'unfashionably' shaped women. Besides, by buying clothes that are dark, all vertical lines and 'correct' fabrics, you succeed merely in drawing attention to the 'shamefulness' of your figure, not in hiding it. Is it any surprise that people seem critical of you, if even you don't think yourself worth adornment?

The following exercise is intended to help improve your confidence in your body and in what you wear, whether you are a size 8 or 38.

Think of the types of clothes you plan to wear when you've been on a diet and lost the desired weight, and write them down. What sort of shapes will suit you best then? What sort of patterns? Do you imagine wearing leggings, tight dresses and plenty of jewellery? Or, like Dorothy, a particular colour:

> Red. Always I think of red. When I'm overweight, I wear black and navy, but when I'm as I imagine I will be, I'm in red, with sheer black stockings, and a close-fitting dress that'll enhance my cleavage. With beads. Definitely, beads. Two, three strands of heavy, bright beads. I've got them in my drawer waiting for the day.

Maybe it's a miniskirt, a cloak, a trouser suit, a comfy, fluffy woollen sweater, a brilliant blue-and-yellow exercise leotard for the aerobics class, a gossamer bikini, a silk nightdress with buttoned-up bits and frilly edges – you know the sorts of things all of us have in mind and picture ourselves wearing, once the diet is over, to the admiration and approval of all concerned.

Now, go out to the shops and BUY SOMETHING ON YOUR LIST, IN YOUR CURRENT SIZE. Don't delay. Don't put it off until your diet's done. You can always get another one then, if it really means that much to you. Leggings? Get a pair that'll fit you, in the colour *you* like best, not the colour which you think will best suit your current weight. Bikini? Get one. Get it by mail order, if you'd rather, and, if you want, get some of those silk night-time thingies at the same time. Don't swamp yourself in some voluminous garment: buy something that fits, clings. If necessary take a friend with you to advise – a kind friend, not the sort who is hung up about fashion and figures.

Now wear it as you would when you are thin: with style and panache, not furtively.

The point is, stop treating your current figure as one not deserving of the best you can give it. OK, so you'd prefer to do all this when you're a size 10, but you're not, and until you get there, stop living in Clothes Limbo.

So, select a day and wear your chosen garment. Go to work in it, to the cinema, fetch the kids in it, wear it at a disco, take it to bed – whatever you like. Just get yourself gradually away from wearing apologetic clothes chosen just to hide your figure, and towards wearing confident, admirable clothes that don't. Make a virtue of your size and shape. It is individuality, not the patsyish struggle for uniformity, that makes a person interesting.

If you're too hard up at the moment to buy something new, form a clothes exchange with some other women, and pool together all the clothes from your wardrobes. Every dieter has clothes that she doesn't wear, probably because they aren't any longer in her size (or will only be so in the dreamy, distant, post-diet future), or that she regards as too risky to wear just yet, and if you get together enough people you're bound to find a rich source of new garments to choose from.

Take Action!

At the back of the book you will find copies of form letters to your local clothes shops, to your MP and to the editor of a women's magazine. Send them off. If you can, get other people to sign, too, turning them into a petition. Make photocopies, and send off several copies to different people. These letters point out the truth about weight and good health, and ask shops and magazines to acknowledge the 50 per cent of women who are size 16+ by improving their range and using models that are other than skeletal to show off the products. Alternatively, you can write your own letter, or add your own comments to the bottom of the given one. But whatever you do, make sure you send something. Not only is it good for your morale, but you'll also be helping to change fashion and thus ease the burden for all women and children. It is incredible how much influence a single letter can have. It takes only one letter to inform an MP that weight is not bad for you and that dieting is. One letter, and we are already one MP better off. The other day a TV advert was banned because thirteen people had complained about it to the advertising authority. As few as thirteen people and an enormously expensive and important ad gets dropped! With just a small amount of effort we, the public, can achieve great results. So, use your power. Cut out, sign, and send the letters off.

The Golden Rules

There are two parts to this plan: Exercise (Chapter 18) and Food (Chapter 19). But first, it is absolutely essential that you read and follow the five golden rules of successful weight loss. They are:

> Rule 1: To Hell with Dieting!
> Rule 2: Be Patient.
> Rule 3: *Don't* Go it Alone.
> Rule 4: Start Healthy.
> Rule 5: Don't Put Your Life on Hold.

Rule 1: To Hell with Dieting! Once you've read these three chapters it's time to choose your D-Day – the day you will say, 'To hell with dieting!' Mark it in your diary as the beginning of the twelve-week period. Due to a bill introduced in the House of Commons, as of 1994, 5 May each year is National No-Diet Day. In choosing your own no-diet day to start on the plan you are not doing something alone, you are joining thousands of other women who after years of being oppressed by dieting and figure concerns are finally saying 'enough is enough'.

Next you must abandon your all-or-nothing attitude to food. Remember you are eating sensibly, not dieting, and so indulging in a Mars Bar is not breaking a diet. Therefore there is no reason to go the whole hog and eat six Mars Bars. Even if you go quite dotty and order a seven-course Indian meal from the local take-away, shut yourself in the bedroom with the TV, and scoff the lot, IT DOESN'T MATTER. (You'll probably get an upset tummy and lose what you put on by another route!) Whenever you stray from healthy eating, regard it as a temporary diversion from the main route, not the end of everything. I find it helps to think of the next twelve weeks as a pleasant car journey, say from London to Oxford. You're tootling merrily along, and will get there in the end, but occasionally you have an almighty urge to go off down a sweet little side road to admire some pigs enjoying a snooze in the sun, or a jolly scarecrow (for pigs and scarecrows, read pizzas, chocolate, walnut whip, etc.) These little diversions slow up the journey, but they're enjoyable while they last and certainly should not be allowed to induce anxiety or guilt.

So, just relax and keep on with the plan. The best way to free yourself from the tyranny of dieting is to see all your past attempts and present weaknesses as *funny*. It helps enormously to get together with a friend and swap dieting absurdities.

Even after you have stopped dieting your dieting attitude to food will linger for a while. To begin with you will probably eat rather more than you should, or alternatively you might, despite yourself, always cut meals short, starve yourself for ages then rush to the kitchen in a furtive eating frenzy. This will pass. Gradually, over the weeks, you will get accustomed to the fact that the changes you are making on this plan will help you much more than any inane calorie-restricting diet, and that is when you will stop letting food rule your life.

Rule 2: Be Patient. *You cannot change your shape overnight, however maniacally you try.* To make any appreciable difference to your body will take weeks. Therefore, the biggest favour you can do yourself is to have patience and, once you have absorbed all the golden rules, simply *forget* about losing weight. The surest way to fail on a diet is to be constantly preoccupied with it – jumping on the scales every hour to see if your six-mile run has taken effect, whipping out the tape measure every morning, and so forth. Therefore, once you have chosen your D-Day, get rid of your weighing scales. Besides, as we have already seen, scales give a poor indication of your shape because muscle weighs quite a bit more than fat: your waistband or a close-fitting pair of trousers will give a more accurate picture of your figure.

The eating plan is arranged over twelve weeks. Sounds like a long time? Well, you have a choice. If you are impatient you will go on the latest crash diet, lose plenty of pounds to begin with, suffer near starvation in the process, and soon put the podge back on again. On average, women do this once a year, year in, year out, from their early teens until their fifties and after, getting gradually fatter in the process. Compared to that, isn't a twelve-week plan a piece of lightning-fast wizardry?

So: learn the rules of the plan, settle your D-Day, and then stop worrying. FORGET about how much weight you want to lose, how many calories that means, and how long it will take.

Rule 3: Don't Go it Alone. One of the main reasons diets fail is because the dieter is isolated – often in a family of hungry men and children. You can't subject them all to 1000 calories a day. Children need a full, fairly rich diet if they are to grow up healthily, and even if your husband needs to lose weight, you'll be luckier than most women if you can get him to do a damn thing about it. I have plenty of friends who force themselves to eat less than a worm, while their blokes, three times their size, guzzle everything in sight. The success rates of diets would be higher if women weren't continually subject to everybody else's (often wilful) attempts to sabotage their efforts. (I can remember one character actually saying to me, 'Come *on*, have a cake. What's in a cake? Only a little butter and sugar.') Even other dieters take a perverse delight in tempting you. It's just not possible for most of us to succeed under such conditions.

'The evening meal should be an exquisite, enjoyable experience,' writes Ann Leader, a researcher whom I quoted earlier. 'How often this is not the case!' she continues, and gives a very memorable picture of how difficult life can be for a woman embarking on a difficult slimming diet:

> The more usual scenario features a tired, tense housewife trying to get the whole sordid affair over as quickly as possible. Her hungry, hassled husband needs an instant food fix. He cannot be deprived of history in the making and so requires peace and solitude when he tunes in compulsively to the 6 o'clock news. The starving hordes of cranky children need to be stuffed with food to ensure their silence and his comfort. The cook is getting more frazzled by the minute

and gulps down any old makeshift meal that comes her way. She contents herself with scraps. After 1 hour, the kitchen glistens, the cherubs sleep and her happy husband, hushed with food, is whistling softly in the shower.

This sad state of affairs could be reversed with a little forward planning. The children could be fed their favourite dinner at 5 o'clock, long before breaking point is reached. Husband could watch his 6 o'clock news free from hustle and bustle of meal time. The cook could treat herself to a relaxing predinner soak in Radox, happy in the knowledge that her modern partner is bonding with and bedding down their cherished offspring. Why should he be deprived of the precious moments!

The happy couple could eat at 8 o'clock, alone and un-interrupted. A microwave helps to complete the miracle!

Going it together is one of the most critical elements of any new eating arrangement; indeed, of almost any change in lifestyle. It is very important to get the cooperation of as many of the people with whom you regularly eat as possible – husbands, lovers, children, flatmates.

One of the great advantages of this plan is that it operates gradually, so making the change shouldn't be difficult. You are not asking all your nearest and dearest to eat a fraction of their normal quantity in order that you can become a waif before summer sets in. You're asking them to eat as much as they like of stuff that's good for them and for you.

The eating plan is structured so that you *gradually* introduce changes to your diet, and thus by the end of the twelve-week period the new way of eating has become your preferred way of eating.

Rule 4: Start Healthy. It seems to be the curse of modern life that 80 per cent of people are tired 80 per cent of the time – I've heard doctors make that comment about their patients more times than I've eaten sticky toffee pudding. It certainly applied to me, and this is why I want to give a brief account of how, corny though it sounds, my life was changed. It happened very recently and it happened overnight. Over two nights to be precise.

For a depressingly large portion of my life I have had very little energy. There were periods, sometimes lasting weeks at a time, when I was so physically drained that I had to do my work lying in bed. Of course, I *could* get up. Indeed I forced myself to do all kinds of things, including trek round India three times. But by and large life was much, much easier lying down. Exercise was hell.

I always took it that that was how I was made. After all, the world seems full of weak and listless people. Nevertheless, it was worrying, particularly when I developed other strange symptoms: depersonalization and panic attacks, and repeated cystitis and thrush.

Then, several years ago, after recovering from a nasty virus I'd caught in Kenya, my condition abruptly worsened threefold. I found I *couldn't* get out of bed, and, more frighteningly, that the lethargy had begun to encroach upon my mind. I couldn't concentrate or work.

'Oh yes,' said my GP breezily, 'post-viral syndrome. It usually goes after a few months.'

'And if it doesn't?' I said in alarm.

'Oh well, then after six months it's classed as ME. The longer it goes on, the harder it is to get rid of.' Such a chirpy, bright-voiced little man.

I was in despair. ME is a devastating illness. I telephoned a local doctor who specializes in allergies and intolerances, though I did so with little hope that she could help me.

After very careful questioning she did two things. She suggested that I was intolerant of certain foods, especially wheat. And, after noting that I had had repeated antibiotics (for cystitis) she suggested I might have a problem with candida in the gut – for which she prescribed an antifungal medicine.

I stopped eating wheat and took the medicine. Exactly two days later I was so full of energy that after two hours of vigorous tennis my thin, fit young partner was begging me to stop. At night I went whizzing round the house, clearing out the attic, while he lay collapsed on the sofa.

I was fortunate in that my problem was easily diagnosed – getting to the root of vague illnesses such as mine can be very difficult. But both wheat intolerance and candida are extremely common. When my doctor suggested that wheat was the culprit, at first I simply could not believe her. How ridiculous, I thought! Only cranky types have trouble with such common foodstuffs. I'd also heard some rubbish (as I thought) about the very things one craves being the culprits. I'd always dismissed that as a hangover of Puritan nonsense. But, lo and behold, what is the only thing I have ever craved? Wheat! And, at the worst moments of my illness I was eating wheat by the barrelful.

Several times since then I've doubted that wheat can really have this effect and gorged on pasta, only to find that two or three days later I am not only lying in defeat on the bed, but am in a depressed, hopeless, almost catatonic state.

Never, never pay attention to anyone, however eminent, when they pooh pooh common foodstuffs as possible causes of illness. Allergies are not in the least bit cranky. Thousands of people suffer dreadful symptoms which they have never connected with such everyday staples as dairy products, sugar, eggs, potatoes, tomatoes and many more.

Candida, too, produces a huge range of symptoms, from loss of libido, through depersonalization to sheer exhaustion, even skin problems. Women who suffer candida in the vagina (thrush) are frequently sufferers; most women have at some time been prescribed antibiotics for cystitis, and antibiotics encourage candida.

So, if you are plagued with symptoms that your doctor can do nothing for, it is worth seeking out an allergy specialist. If this is beyond your means, there are now scores of books on the subject available not only at bookshops but also at health-food stores. Maggie discovered by simple trial and error that the agonizing breast pains she suffered every period ceased completely when she stopped eating cheese at that time of the month.

My simple discovery changed my life. I only wish I'd known it thirty years ago.

Rule 5: Don't Put Your Life on Hold. The easiest way to forget that you wish to lose weight is to start living your life to the full NOW. Wear attractive clothes that *fit*. Living for now also means doing everything that you envisaged doing once you were thin: whether it's a beach holiday, a new haircut, joining a dance class or whatever. Try to get rid of the slimming mentality, which assumes that as soon as you've got yourself into a size 10 or 12 everything will be rosy. Let me tell you: nothing will change unless you change it now. Perhaps if you are a size 26 and unhappy with it, and intend to get down to a size 12, your life might alter dramatically. But for most women being a size 10 does not mean everlasting happiness, love, stability, financial success and weekly holidays in the Caribbean. Far more dreams are realized by virtue of confidence and immediate action than ever by the fact of a featherweight body. And if you're going to be bloody-minded and argue that your self-esteem *depends* on a featherweight body, then think of it this way: you *will* lose weight, so why not borrow a bit of future self-confidence to get you along now?

One of the defining characteristics of a dieter is that she rarely believes the praise of anybody else, and always criticizes herself with extreme harshness, knowing the 'faults' of every separate inch of her body. Next time your partner or family tell you that you do not need to lose weight, pay them the compliment of believing them. Get into the habit of responding to other people, and out of the habit of thinking they must be mentally deficient not to understand.

If, on the other hand, your family and friends tend to be nasty about your weight, give as good as you get. It is absolutely nobody else's business to tell you to lose weight. Yet it is a curious phenomenon that liberal-minded individuals who would not dream of making racist, anti-semitic or sexist remarks, apparently think it quite acceptable to be extremely unpleasant about someone else's figure. It's up to all of us – fat and thin – to show up these discrepancies whenever we hear them. Next time some 'well-meaning' busybody tells you to lose weight, respond pleasantly with an equally intimate comment about their hair, their bad temper or their taste in clothes. At a dinner party recently a scrawny, precisely dressed, genteel woman leaned across to the decidedly plump hostess and recommended, in an audible whisper, a new diet. It was embarrassing and extremely rude. But the hostess was up to it, and retorted aloud: 'How very interesting. I'll exchange it for a tip on how to cure discoloured teeth.'

If your boyfriend is snide and critical, ditch him. You deserve better.

Stop thinking of yourself as a fat person (you probably aren't anyway). That means you must never put yourself down, make jokes about your size, or allow other people to do so. It's very true that people judge you by your own evaluation of yourself. Therefore, making jokes – or excuses – about your size will simply give the message that it is something that *needs* excusing.

14
Calculating Your BMI and WHR Numbers

G et out your tape measure and calculator, go to the bathroom, lock the door and take off your clothes.

The BMI number, as I mentioned in Chapter 4, is your Body Mass Index number. This is a measure of weight that is widely used by insurance companies as a measure of your health, and to help them calculate premiums on life insurance policies. Their estimate of what your BMI number should be forms the basis for many of the important modern height–weight charts. The second number is your Waist-to-Hip Ratio. This is a much more important measurement which I also introduced earlier, in Chapter 5.

In the meantime, however, find the scales and stand on them.

Calculating Your BMI Number

This calculation requires only two measurements: your weight (in kilograms) and your height (in metres). Since you're supposed to be measuring your body weight and not the weight of your shoes and clothes, it's best to weigh yourself naked and measure your height without heels. Your BMI number is then calculated by dividing your weight by the square of your height, or

$$BMI = weight/height^2$$

If your maths isn't that hot, then the way to do this is to divide your weight by your height, twice. Type in your weight (in kilograms). Press '÷'. Type in your height (in metres). Press '÷' again. Type in your height a second time. Press '='. The result is your BMI number.

For example:

The Queen of Sheba weighs 71.8 kg, and she's 1.65 m tall. Her BMI number is therefore: $71.8 \div 1.65 \div 1.65 = 26.4$

In case you've got a pair of scales that measures only in pounds and a tape measure that uses only inches, then do the calculation as described (i.e. divide your weight in pounds by your height in inches, twice) and multiply the result by 705.

For example:

The Queen of Sheba weighs 11 st 4 lbs, which is 158 lbs. She is 5 ft 5 ins tall, which is 65 ins. Her BMI number is therefore: $158 \div 65 \div 65 \times 705 = 26.4$

Naturally, the number you get will vary when your weight varies. For women this is particularly important, since several physiological factors influence our weight – the menstrual cycle, pregnancy, lactation and the menopause. However, if you are an adult woman, the likelihood is that your BMI number will be somewhere between 19 and 30. If you're within that range, then, as I explained in Chapter 5, providing you are not apple-shaped, the most up-to-date medical research shows that your weight will have no influence on your health or life-expectancy.

For me, at 5 ft 9 ins, that means I could weigh anything between 52 kg (9 st 6 lbs) and 92 kg (14 st 8 lbs).

If you find yourself exclaiming in disbelief, then go back to Chapter 5 and read it again.

If your BMI number is below 19 you are probably medically underweight. I say 'probably' because every woman's body is different: for a few it is healthy to be so light, for most it is definitely unhealthy. If you are below 18, you are definitely underweight, and ought to start eating more. Below 17 and you're heading into the anorexic range.

At the other end, if you are over 30, then you are significantly overweight. Providing, however, you take regular exercise and your hips are larger than your waist (see the next exercise) then, with the exception of possible joint trouble, your weight is nothing much to worry about as far as health is concerned. If your BMI is much above 30 – say, over 35 – then you are definitely overweight (it is, after all, hard to be that heavy and still be pear-shaped) and from the health point of view you ought to do something about it. Once more, however, regular exercise and healthy eating will do you much more good than a strict reducing diet.

I repeat, this information is taken from the best medical evidence.

For height (without shoes)		Weights for different BMI values stone (kilograms)					
ft in	m	BMI = 20		BMI = 25		BMI = 30	
4 10	1.47	6.11	(43.2)	8.7	(54)	10.3	(64.8)
4 11	1.5	7.1	(45)	8.12	(56.3)	10.9	(67.5)
5 0	1.52	7.4	(46.2)	9.1	(57.6)	10.12	(69.3)
5 1	1.55	7.8	(48.1)	9.6	(60.1)	11.5	(72.1)
5 2	1.57	7.10	(49.3)	9.10	(61.6)	11.9	(73.9)
5 3	1.6	8.1	(51.2)	10.1	(64)	12.1	(76.8)
5 4	1.63	8.5	(53.1)	10.6	(66.4)	12.7	(79.7)
5 5	1.65	8.8	(54.5)	10.10	(68.1)	12.12	(81.7)
5 6	1.68	8.12	(56.4)	11.1	(70.6)	13.4	(84.7)
5 7	1.7	9.1	(57.8)	11.5	(72.3)	13.9	(86.7)
5 8	1.73	9.6	(59.9)	11.11	(74.8)	14.2	(89.9)
5 9	1.75	9.9	(61.3)	12.1	(76.6)	14.6	(91.9)
5 10	1.78	9.13	(63.4)	12.6	(79.2)	14.13	(95.1)
5 11	1.8	10.3	(64.8)	12.10	(81)	15.4	(97.2)
6 0	1.83	10.7	(67)	13.2	(83.7)	15.11	(100.5)
6 1	1.85	10.11	(68.5)	13.6	(85.6)	16.2	(102.7)
6 2	1.88	11.2	(70.7)	13.13	(88.4)	16.9	(106)
6 3	1.91	11.7	(73)	14.5	(91.2)	17.3	(109.4)
6 4	1.93	11.10	(74.5)	14.9	(93.1)	17.8	(111.7)

The numbers tabulated above apply to both adult men and adult women of all frame sizes. This is not to say that all bodies have the same structure, but that the BMI is a crude means of determining healthy weight ranges and that it therefore does not possess the power to make such narrow distinctions. Naturally, however, one would expect that a woman of a given size would weigh less than a man of equal height. You will also see in the table that the range given is quoted to the nearest 100 g and to the nearest pound; but, again, this is not to be taken too seriously. These figures represent those weights corresponding to BMI = 20, 25 and 30. The precision is a consequence of applying a strict formula, not an indication that our health is dependent on the minutest variations in weight.

Calculating Your Waist-to-Hip Ratio

It is simple to calculate your WHR. All you have to do is divide your waist measurement by your hip measurement. Because of this, it doesn't matter what units you use – centimetres or inches, it makes no difference, providing you are consistent and use the same units for each measurement.

Standing upright (to do this accurately it is best to be watching yourself in the mirror) you need to measure your waist at the level of your belly button, and your hips at the top of the hip bone.

Now divide your waist measurement by your hip measurement. For example:

The Queen of Sheba's waist is 26 ins and her hips are 35 ins. Therefore her Waist-to-Hip Ratio is: WHR = 26 ÷ 35 = 0.74

This number tells you, from the clinical point of view, whether you are an apple or a pear shape. You're probably thinking that you could have figured that out without resorting to mathematics, but, as with the BMI number, the WHR number provides an objective medical judgement not a subjective one. And from the medical point of view the division between apple-shaped and pear-shaped which is different for women and men, is as follows:

	Women WHR	Men WHR
pear shape	less than 0.8	less than 0.9
apple shape	more than 0.8	more than 0.9

If you're pear-shaped, then you're in good shape. If you're much into the apple-shaped range, through having a lot of surplus weight around your abdomen, then it's a good idea to get it off. If you are thin already and apple-shaped, then don't worry about it. That's probably the way you're meant to be, and, as far as you

241

are concerned, there's absolutely nothing unhealthy about it.

For an average woman, the healthiest way to be, if such a precise statement must be made, is a stone or two above the figure given for her height on most height–weight charts, and pear-shaped. Note that I refer to 'the average woman'. I'll say it again: every woman's body is different. If you are naturally of a different shape and weight when eating healthily and keeping fit, then that is the best way for you to be. In spite of what almost all of the popular diet books still tell you, there is no such thing as a single 'ideal' weight (or weight range) for every woman of a given height.

On average, women tend to have a WHR between 0.7 and 1; and men, between 0.75 and 1.1. Again, for women, the value will tend to vary according to the time of the month. Also, of course, it won't work if you're pregnant.

There! That's it. You've just mastered the two most important equations in the study of the relationship between weight and health.

How Often Should You Take Your BMI and WHR Measurements on the Plan?

As often as you want. You don't have to take them at all. I've written this chapter primarily as a matter of interest. If you find it encouraging (as I sometimes do) to chart the way your BMI and WHR vary over the twelve weeks, then I suggest taking one set of measurements the day you begin, another halfway through, and a third at the end.

Proceed . . .

15

Exercise

There is no getting round it: if you want to lose weight you absolutely *must* exercise.

Don't groan and moan. If a lifelong couch potato like myself can start enjoying exercise, *anybody* can. The trick is to realize that exercise does not have to be half an hour of crashingly boring exercises each morning.

Experts often puzzle over the fact that although, by and large, we eat very much less today than we used to 100 years ago, we're actually heavier. If you look at the quantity of food the Victorian rich tucked into, it's surprising they weren't all balloon-shaped. Various theories have been dreamed up to account for this – one I came across suggested intriguingly that as pollutants collect in human fat cells in preference to vital organs, fat has become a necessary adaptation to a polluted world. True or not, one of the main reasons for the discrepancy is that, in the olden days, people of *all* classes took a great deal more exercise than most of us today.

For centuries, horses and feet were the only ready means of transport: the diary of any nineteenth-century gentleman makes frequent reference to ten-mile walks and three-day horseback outings. Throughout history, women without servants have had the physically demanding jobs of laundry, scrubbing, shopping and even fetching water from the well. Doctors and clergymen in country parishes habitually walked or rode miles each day from village to village, and their patients and congregations likewise would travel miles to visit them – even as recently as the 1950s.

The chapter on exercise in *The Art of Beauty*, by the Toilet Specialist, reveals that even society women frequently tramped ten to fifteen miles across the moors between lunch and dinner. Lawn tennis and golf were both recommended as perfectly suitable pastimes for women, and 'cricket is so much played at girls' schools and colleges nowadays'. The author also explains that 'Gymnastics are perhaps better calculated to develop the figure, and bestow a

243

graceful carriage than any other form of exercise'. Female gym-
nasts even wore Victorian versions of the garb women wear in
aerobics classes today: a tight-fitting combination garment, loose
full knickerbockers of serge or flannel reaching to two or three
inches below the knee, and low-heel, canvas shoes.

Before we discuss the different types of modern exercise I am
going to show you that there are far greater incentives for a bit of
hop and jiggle than simply the prospect of losing weight. It is now
known that the most efficient way to stay younger and active all
your life is to exercise. There are 7000 people in Britain today
over 100 years old – why not try and join them?

If the thought of such antiquity doesn't appeal, at least the
prospect of a healthy active retirement ought to, however long
you have to put up with it!

Exercise is not only good for weight loss, it is the best possible
way to keep yourself youthful.

Exercise keeps you looking young. It keeps your muscles strong,
bones dense, ligaments tight, stamina high, body supple, immune
system effective. It improves mood and lowers stress. Regular exercise protects against heart disease. It can make your heart and
lungs over ten years younger by maximizing your lung capacity.
Also, by improving circulation, exercise keeps the brain well oxy-
genated, thus ensuring the preservation of brain cells as you grow
older. Another of the ways in which we age is by converting muscle
into fat. So, although you may not put on weight as you grow
older, unless you exercise you will probably become fatter. 'Everything that gets worse as you get older, gets better as you exercise,'
says a researcher quoted in *Health and Fitness* magazine.

Combined with healthy eating, exercise will keep your body
working at maximum efficiency, and your energy and spirits high.
As I showed earlier, lack of fitness is much more detrimental to
your health than even a substantial amount of excess weight.

One of the overwhelming benefits of exercise is that it also gives
you an incentive to get on and do things. This is particularly
helpful for people who, like me, have sedentary jobs. I used to
have the greatest difficulty getting round to anything that wasn't
already part of my routine – be it nasty jobs like clearing out the
attic and writing letters, or even pleasant things like making
the effort to go to the theatre, or visiting friends who live in
inconvenient places.

I decided to start exercising, and began by doing forty minutes every other day. I soon changed it to forty minutes every day, which I found much easier to keep up, simply because it quickly became a habit like brushing one's teeth. Now, whenever I get back from my tennis, squash or whatever, I'm in a good mood to get on with other useful jobs that I had previously ignored.

Also, contrary to the popular belief that exercise increases your appetite, I find it dramatically reduces mine, in particular for the two hours immediately afterwards.

Now we come to weight loss. It's often said that exercise is a lousy way to lose weight because you have to use up 3500 calories to lose one measly pound of fat, and 3500 calories is a crushing amount of jogging and arm-waving. I remember when I was about twenty and my best friend and I were sharing a flat together. One evening, after ten days of rigid dieting, we gave in and gobbled a whole chocolate cake. As the last crumbs disappeared we were overtaken by terrible guilt: there was nothing for it but to exercise the calories away. We put on Queen's *Killer Queen* (over and over again) and danced maniacally until dawn, stopping every half hour to ask each other: 'D'you think the calories are gone yet?' We could not walk for a week afterwards.

Looked at like that, yes, exercise is pretty useless. But that's just one day. I look at it like this. An hour's walking uses up 200–300 calories, which is the equivalent of a light lunch. If, in your old dieting days, you'd missed lunch every day for several weeks you'd expect to see good weight loss. And that is, in effect, what you are doing, only you are having the pleasure of your lunch and the benefits of the walk. In other words, *exercise soon mounts up.*

There are two other critical points to be made about exercise, weight loss and your figure:

1) Regular exercise builds up muscle and thereby increases your basic metabolic rate. This means that you burn up more energy and lose fat. So even though it takes a fair amount of exercise to burn up calories *directly, indirectly* regular exercise leads to more fat loss than those miserable calculations would lead you to believe.

2) Not only is muscle more metabolically active than fat, it also (as you should know by now if you read Part One) weighs more. But Don't Panic! To begin with, as you replace fat with muscle you will not lose much weight. Shock, horror: you might even gain some! But you *will* get thinner (remember my experience in the gym?). Muscle is denser than fat. A pound of muscle occupies less space than a pound of fat. So when you replace a pound of fat

with a pound of muscle, you lose girth. As you get further into the plan, however, you will start to lose excess weight as well.

Which Exercise?

Begin by asking yourself the following questions:

1) Do you prefer the heat or the cool? Being too hot or too cold is one of the important reasons we get fed up with exercise. I suffer most dreadfully with the heat: my face looks like a boiled lobster and my energy levels plummet. I hated tennis all the years I had to play it at school for the simple reason that we only ever played it in the summer term, but now, as soon as summer is well and truly over, I join the tennis club. First, it's cheaper; second, the courts are always free; and third, however chilly it is to start, you quickly warm up and thereafter remain at a comfortable temperature. I simply can't understand those loonies who play in high summer . . .

Conversely, those of you who suffer in the cold may try squash or badminton.

If, like me, you have strong views about temperature you may need to do different kinds of exercise in summer and in winter. I adore walking in the rain (winter exercise) and in summer plunge into the swimming pool.

2) Do you have bits that wobble? If the answer's yes, then don't go for the sport that's going to exacerbate them, such as jogging. Bosoms and bottoms can play merry and painful hell with one's good sporting intentions. If you are well endowed, swimming's a very good bet, at least until you lose some weight. In fact, just as you may need to alter your exercise summer and winter, so you may need to begin on one kind and when you are thinner progress to another. Too often people feel they have to pick their sport and stick to it willy nilly. Actually it should be like a good-fitting dress: tailor-made for your particular needs at any one time.

3) Do you know that there are more than 19 million sports injuries a year? It's true, so don't overdo the exercise. This boring piece of advice is trotted out in every exercise book, and most people in their first flush of enthusiasm ignore it at their peril. Let me just say that when I first joined a gym I didn't take the trouble to warm up properly. This caused my knee to get injured on the rowing machine, which put me out of action for two months

and which I can still feel three years later. Sports injuries really are no joke, but can be very simply avoided. Always follow the expert's instructions.

4) How many sports can you name? There are countless sports and activities I haven't mentioned, and the place to find out about them is your local library. You'll be surprised how many things are on offer, and the people who attend, being amateurs and eager to attract recruits, will probably be friendly to work with, as well as providing the team spirit that will encourage you to keep it up. I know many people who've made very good friends by joining local sports groups.

5) Do you have somebody who would be fun to play with? (And I don't mean some awfully earnest twit who likes to boost his/her ego at your expense.) In partner sports, you've got to find a compatible person to play with: not only one of roughly your own standard, but one who takes it as seriously or unseriously as you do. There's little worse than playing with someone who regards the game as a battle ground of exertion and humourlessness.

6) Do you realize how quickly you will improve? This is a piece of good cheer. I used to think that it took years of dedication to notice an improvement in one's fitness levels, but in fact it happens very quickly indeed. The one occasion when I kept up the dreaded jogging for three weeks I was amazed to find that I noticed an improvement in *days*.

All in all, it doesn't matter how you do your exercise, as long as you do it regularly and keep it up for thirty to sixty minutes at least three times a week. (A book I have found very useful in getting you off to a good start is *Eat Yourself Thin*, by Arabella Melville and Colin Johnson.) Last but not least, it's absolutely true that after exercise your brain releases endorphins, chemicals that make you feel good. I was astonished to find just how good life seems after half an hour of vigorous activity. This may not happen your first day, but it will sooner or later. So whenever the prospect of exercise depresses you, remember how jolly you will feel afterwards.

Exercise is always talked about as if the scores of different activities it includes – working out at a gym, playing tennis, jogging, walking the dog, splashing around in a river and larking about in a field – all felt the same, and were all equally loathsome. But exercise varies wildly in what it feels like, and once you begin to see it as a range of activities which includes everything from the po-faced agonies endured by over-muscled young men in the gym to the raucous pleasure of a game of hide and seek, it quickly loses its power to depress you.

Jogging is, in my opinion, the vilest of the lot. Unfortunately it's the one that so many people begin with – on several memorable occasions I've dutifully donned tracksuit and set off gasping and wobbling round the block for what seemed like half an hour at least, only to find I had been gone all of four minutes. Jogging may be cheap and comparatively easy, and perhaps eventually one can learn to love it, but for most of us it's boring and, unless you have proper training and expensive shoes, bad for your joints. Added to which, if you've got any sort of bosom or bottom it's painful and you attract unwelcome attention from men who yell at you out of cars. For this last reason I always used to go jogging at night, and thus in fear of my life (female joggers have been the target of some nasty attacks, so if you do jog make very, very sure you go in safe places). Better still, learn self-defence. So – unless you really love it – to hell with jogging.

Walking is much more civilized, and it is a good idea to get out of the habit of taking the car everywhere and use your legs instead. To do any real good you need to walk for twenty minutes three times a week at a pace that leaves you slightly out of breath but not gasping. A good test is whether you can sing: if you're too puffed to warble, then you're overdoing things. Walking, especially in cool, damp weather, is also marvellous for the complexion. If you find it dull, get a Walkman: you can listen to music or even learn a language. I read recently some good advice to walkers, namely that on each walk you should look out for one particular thing: interesting chimney pots, different types of tree, etc.

Swimming is, without doubt, one of the star forms of exercise, not least because it strains no part of your anatomy. The water resistance quickly builds strength in places that often don't get used, like shoulders, inner thighs and arms. It's excellent for very hefty people (no wobbling bottom or bosom) and also for older, disabled or chronically sedentary people. Swimming has one other absolutely marvellous advantage, namely that even when pounding along briskly for half an hour without stopping I never encountered that awful gasping and wheezing that comes with thirty seconds of running.

The drawback of swimming is finding a convenient pool. I'm

also a coward about cold water, but a few lengths quickly warms one up. It is a huge advantage that it is virtually impossible to get too hot. If you get tired of doing lengths you can try diving or learn a new stroke. Then there are the endless games you can invent, especially if you bring along a friend or two plus a large ball. (One good one that gets the arm muscles working is to sit on the ball, clutching it between your bottom and your calves, and to try to propel yourself the length of the pool while remaining upright. If you have a race like this it's unlikely you'll reach the end without hysterical laughter, because people look so silly doing it.)

Cycling is marvellous for the legs, and very exhilarating all round, so long as you are brave on the roads. I used to cycle about town until I bought a motorcar and saw from the driver's point of view just how hair-raising bicycling in traffic can be. So, as a motorist, let me take this opportunity to get on my soap box: GET GOOD LIGHTS ON YOUR BICYCLE. Many cyclists seem to think lights are an optional extra, and evidently don't realize just how frighteningly difficult it is for a motorist to see a cyclist in the dusk or dark, even up close.

The Toilet Specialist is particularly keen on cycling, and indeed the 1890s saw a massive craze for the sport, with crowds gathering in Battersea Park to cheer on the cyclists. But, she warns coyly, this should be indulged in only in the very *strictest* moderation by teenage girls, because 'the pressure of even the most satisfactory of saddles is largely exerted upon the very portions of their physical structure which should be left most free to grow and expand in the way Nature intended'. Make what you will of that!

Tennis is enjoyable, even if you've never picked up a racket in your life. If you can't afford lessons, try arranging a swop with a friend who plays well – you teach her driving/knitting/electronics/Mexican cookery or do a spot of babysitting. If you still can't get lessons, just grab a partner and bash the ball back and forth. You'll no doubt get some snooty looks from real tennis players, but who cares? My partner and I have invented our own game, which takes absolutely no account of lines on the court, is three times as energetic as the average game and twenty times more fun, at least for those who aren't any good at tennis proper. In my experience, serious tennis players are much more concerned that you turn up looking reasonably neat (either wearing white, or at least a tracksuit) than about how you play. Oh, and if you're a beginner bring plenty of balls or you'll spend all day running after those you've missed.

Squash has a rather male image: one thinks of a fat balding businessman stripping off and thwacking a ball about in an attempt to show that he has more machismo than his partner. The nice thing about squash is that you're alone on the court with your partner (plenty of romantic possibilities) and not (like swimming or jogging) likely to be bashed into by some stray lout.

And now we come to gyms. Not so long ago the very word 'gym' filled me with *gloom*, but I've now discovered that they are actually one of the more pleasant ways to exercise. You don't get the nice views and country air, of course, but the machines these days have interesting graphics to spur you on. Also, on a properly devised routine you change machines frequently in order to exercise all the different muscle groups.

Socially, gyms can also be nice to visit. You'll feel as embarrassed as hell on your first day, but you quickly find that nobody looks at you or makes you feel fat/shy/odd/wobbly/out of place since they're all even odder shapes than you are. You can meet and talk to other people, and some gyms have a café or bar as well. A good gym will do you a proper set of fitness tests, work out a personal routine and show you how to use the machines so you won't hurt yourself or turn into one of those misshapen hulks you occasionally see barging down the street. The disadvantage, of course, is that they are expensive, although some let you pay week by week. On the other hand, if you've paid there is an incentive to get your money's worth.

Exercising at home to a video is as boring as ... gosh, I don't know what's as boring as doing that. I can never understand how anybody manages to stick at it for long, although my aunt lost her 5 st with the help of this method. I had some success when I put my exercise bicycle in front of the TV. Another time I tried painting at the same time, with interesting results. Anything so long as the work-out is enjoyable, not a trial of endurance and a test of floorboard strength.

Conserving canals for the National Trust, digging a new plot in the garden, taking part in mock battles with English Heritage, researching diet books in a multistorey library, joining an angry demonstration, starting a riot – all marvellous forms of exercise.

Then there are also the silly sports. For example, taking one dog and one or more friends, play Doggy in the Middle with a ball or frisbee. Most dogs are very obliging, though I suspect my mother's two tubby little pugs Bertie and Harry would find it uphill work. If you can bear the embarrassment of being mistaken for an American college student, play frisbee on your own. Or how about football with the children? Anything will do as long as you have to exert yourself a bit and get your heartbeat going and your arms and legs waving. Remember, thirty to sixty minutes three or four times a week, and you've done all that's required of you. Newsagents and toyshops are filled with wonderful collections of inexpensive games, bats and balls. Last summer I bought two 'badminton' rackets for £1.50 and had a delightful and very strenuous time bashing the infernal shuttlecock about in a high wind. I also have in my garden a £12 toy called 'swingball'. This consists of a metal stick you poke into the ground, with a ball on a long string attached to it. The idea is to thwack the ball about with the bats provided: best played when sozzled, absolutely terrifying if played at high speed!

Skipping is very good exercise, though extraordinarily hard to do if you are no longer a schoolgirl. Discos are good exercise, and ballroom dancing, tap dancing, barn dancing, square dancing. I like to jiggle round the house with the record player on, dusting. It cheers you up as well.

16

The Food Plan

There is a particular sort of person I most dislike:

She is fearfully healthy. She is lean, even sinewy, and quite likely sports a suntan. She bashes off about how she loves fresh fruit and vegetables, and oil-free salads adorned by those horrid little things which sprout pale protuberances in dark cupboards. She never looks at a squidgy cake or creamy thing – indeed these make her feel positively faint – and as for sugar, *well!* Oh, and she's not to keen on booze either, but I dare say she sips little quantities of white wine at her elegant lunches now and then. She wrinkles early.

These sort of people are not part of real life, though tiresomely common on TV and grinning at you from the bookshop window. They make the silly mistake that whatever odd regime has worked for them *must* work for everyone else, when the truth is that individuals vary hugely in their make-up. These diet gurus are also far too extreme in their efforts to convert us. We buy their books intending to start afresh, but find we simply cannot face such radical changes. The book gets dumped out of sight; we return to our old habits, but now feeling guilty as well.

It *is* possible to change your eating habits – and change them dramatically – but it can't be done overnight. My plan spreads it gently over twelve weeks. It worked for me and, believe me, I was a hardened case. For example: butter wasn't butter unless it was spread an inch thick. I had such a passion for creamy cheesy sauce that I poured it on everything – fish, fowl and four-footed beast; even on curry! Food was not worth the effort of conveying it to my mouth unless it was hot and squidgy (salads absolutely beneath contempt). I succeeded in changing my eating habits by making gradual changes. I succeeded so well, in fact, that I find I cannot stomach the old stuff.

You should think of the plan not as something you impose upon your ordinary way of life, but a means of adapting your ordinary

252

way of living so that it is the best possible one for your health and your weight. If you really have to lose weight quickly, for whatever reason, then my plan doesn't prevent you from doing so.

So What Is a Healthy Diet, Then?

There is a basic standard of nutrition that we all need. A healthy diet should not focus on one particular type of food, should aim to be low in sugars (but by no means exclude them altogether), high in fresh fruit and vegetables and fibre (but not to the excesses proposed in *The F-Plan Diet*) and low in fats, particularly animal fats (but not to the extreme degree suggested in *The Hip and Thigh Diet* and its ilk).

See?

End of healthy-eating lecture.

Weight-Loss Tips

For those of you who want to enhance the weight-loss effects of the plan, there are three tips worth bearing in mind.

1) Eat little and often – grazing, as it's called by trendy people. Remember Nanny's exhortation to the children, 'Don't eat between meals or you'll spoil your appetite'? Nannies are *always* right and regular snacks even on fruit and raw vegetables will go a surprising way to fill you up. The worst thing you can do, both physically and psychologically, is starve yourself all day and then eat one big meal. If you aim to go no longer than four hours without food you'll keep your metabolism ticking over efficiently.

2) Henceforth there will be no such thing as 'treats'. Labelling things as treats makes them twice as desirable as they actually are. If you simply must have (for example) chocolate, have it. Don't feel guilty – really enjoy each mouthful. If you are the kind of person who functions on rewards, try to make them non-edible: a bottle of scent, a book or item of clothing.

3) Aim to eat your last meal at least three or four hours before you go to bed. This way the calories will be less likely to be stored as fat.

To Booze or Not to Booze?

A healthy diet should also be a low-alcohol one. Alcohol is full of calories. What's more, regular drinkers are more apt to become the dreaded apple-shape so injurious to health. But this is the bit that I've never managed to do. I like booze, always have, and every attempt I've ever made to cut it out has failed. This does not mean I'm about to put you on a high-alcohol diet, only that changes in your life must be realistic. I take heart from the fact that, increasingly the ill effects of alcohol seem to have been overrated, and that the cookery writer John Tovey consumes ten glasses of wine a day and still lost three stone.

If you are a regular drinker it's worth making an effort to switch to one of the less calorific tipples. White wine is the best of these, although a year ago I couldn't touch the stuff – I thought it thin and nauseating. But I persevered, sampling in particular the delicious New Zealand and Australian wines, and now the mere sight of any other kind of alcohol gives me a hangover. Moral: you'll be amazed at your taste buds' adaptability.

The difficulty of alcohol is that, unlike other types of sustenance, there's no substitute for the lift it gives you. (*Don't* be tempted to take up smoking: it's a hundred times worse for you than several stone of fat.) If intoxication is what you're after you'll soon pick up tricks to make a little alcohol have a large effect, such as sipping slowly and not drinking your ration on a full stomach. I tend to do my best writing late at night and thus need something to help me unwind before going to sleep. I found that by the simple expedient of eating earlier in the evening (which is recommended anyway) I was able to halve my wine intake without losing the relaxing effect.

The Eating Plan

The nutritional part of this plan consists in making six major changes to your diet over a period of twelve weeks. These are, in order:

1) Eating more salads.
2) Eating more fresh fruit and vegetables.
3) Eating more fibre.

4) Cutting down on saturated fats.
5) Cutting down on the amount of oil used in frying.
6) Cutting down on sugar.

That's it. Just six changes and you're home and dry. Introduce them one by one, leaving two weeks in between. At the end of the two-week period the adaptation will have begun to be part of your normal routine, and so it's time to go on to the next step. Obviously, don't give up on the earlier changes to your diet once the two weeks are over. These adjustments are to be adopted for good.

If you are still having difficulty accepting one of the changes after a fortnight, then extend the time. It's important that you consolidate your gains before going on to the next step.

Don't worry about whether or not the rest of what you eat is correct or not. The nature of the plan ensures that will take care of itself.

Weeks one and two: *Eating more salads.* If you want to learn to love salads, you *must* have a delicious dressing. Be stingy in this department (some spartan diet writers deny it altogether) and you might as well give up the attempt. So, if you're not a natural salad lover, begin by using oodles of the stuff: what might have been a paltry, crunchy mass of watery leaves instantly becomes a delicious, filling, nutritious pleasure. Once you've learned to enjoy the salads for themselves you'll find you want to be less lavish with the dressing. For those really keen on losing weight, John Tovey makes the canny point that if the start of your salad is well oiled you don't really mind running out of dressing towards the end.

Commercially prepared dressings are pretty awful. Make it your task this week to devise two really delicious fresh ones. My own absolute favourite is heaps of crushed garlic, natural sea salt, freshly ground black pepper and three or four spoons of oil to one of vinegar. It really pays to get the best quality ingredients you can afford, and in the oil department extra virgin cold pressed olive oil is king. Olive oil is also healthy, being high in unsaturated fats: Mediterranean countries, which use it as their staple source of fat, also suffer from much less heart disease, probably because of it. Good supermarkets nowadays stock a wide range of other interesting oils such as sesame, walnut, hazelnut, which you can use alone or add to ordinary sunflower oil.

Never, never use malt vinegar: that's for fish and chips. Wine, cider and sherry vinegars are delicious, though still not a patch on the pure, delicately sweet bliss of balsamic vinegar (expensive but it lasts for ages). I am in complete agreement with Georgie, who became so attached to balsamic that she claims the whole of her healthy-eating habits and the resulting weight loss, was dependent on this one vital ingredient:

> I dream of writing a book on the subject: *The Balsamic Vinegar Diet*. Balsamic vinegar comes from Italy. It's a very dark, rich, sweet, absolutely scrumptious vinegar that you can almost drink neat from the bottle. It's quite expensive, but you don't need very much of it to turn an ordinary vinaigrette into a heavenly dressing. I reckon a quarter-litre bottle lasts me about three weeks and costs about two pounds. Put in about a teaspoon with a good few glugs of olive oil or, better still, extra virgin olive oil, a clove of garlic, salt and pepper, and you're in heaven. It's a completely different experience from the measly old vegetable oil and wine vinegar stuff you usually get.

If you feel – as I used to – that a meal isn't fit for humans unless it's hot, then make up your usual salady stuff and add to it any of the following: chicken livers, bacon, cut-up and microwaved chicken tikka, tuna and sweetcorn, pepperoni sausage, salami, grilled sweet peppers, hard-boiled egg, fried potatoes, croûtons, sizzling strips of chicken breast, etc., etc. For real hardened anti-cold-food bigots there are even hot dressings. For example: gently cook some diced streaky bacon in a little olive oil for about ten minutes, adding some garlic about a minute before the end. Pour this over a salad of cos lettuce, hard-boiled egg and herbs. Then heat a tablespoon of vinegar in the pan and pour that over, too. Eat.

For these first two weeks it's worth visiting one of the really big supermarket branches, because there you will find an abundant variety of salad ingredients. My local one now stocks twelve varieties of lettuce. Other excellent salad ingredients are fresh spinach leaves, watercress, mustard and cress, spring onions, avocado, carrots, cabbage, fennel, cauliflower florets, nuts, fruit and virtually any herb you care to mention.

Salads are quick, easy to make, can be used either as an accompaniment or as a main course, and are endlessly variable.

You save on time and electricity/gas: there's no planning ahead and putting things in the oven for hours before hand.

If you have trouble getting children to accept salads, a marvellous incentive is to get them growing their own: tomatoes will flourish in gardens, window boxes, grow-bags, pots and even hanging baskets. Picking my own tomatoes from beneath the divinely scented tomato leaves is one of my greatest pleasures.

Weeks three and four: *Eating more fresh fruit and vegetables.* This, of course, began when you increased the amount of salad you ate in weeks one and two. The most obvious way to start is to have fruit for pudding, fresh or in fruit salads. Confirmed anti-fruiters can be seduced with added ice cream or custard until they get a taste for the fruit itself. Try mixing fresh fruit salad with a little tinned fruit in syrup (guava juice is very successful). Adding a shot of liqueur such as Cointreau peps it up no end.

If you have cereal or porridge in the morning, slice some fresh fruit on the top. Pears and apples go well with cheese; Parma ham, with melon.

It is a useful habit to eat oranges, apples, bananas, kiwi fruit, or whatever, as snacks throughout the day, thus staving off hunger and preventing you from overeating when the main meal arrives.

Vegetables do wonderful things for your body, and every meal should have a good supply, as fresh and as lightly cooked as possible to reduce mineral loss. I find piles of raw carrots, celery, peppers and such like unpalatable unless they're dipped in blue cheese dressing or taramasalata. Avocado spread on bread or crackers makes a delicious alternative to butter.

Try cooking with a wok. Using a little oil, and a very high heat for a short space of time, this is a convenient way to cook firm, healthy vegetables. When I first began to stir fry I'd cook the vegetables until they wilted, but most really need only a minute or two to be at their best.

Steaming vegetables improves the flavour and preserves the quality. It took me about four weeks to go from heaps of melted butter on my greens to preferring soy sauce as a dressing.

Weeks five and six: *Eating more fibre.* Dietary fibre is a complex carbohydrate that is not digested by the body and is found in two forms: soluble and insoluble. Kidney beans are high in soluble fibre, while wheat-bran and the skins of peas and sweetcorn are high in insoluble fibre. On average we eat about $^3/_4$ oz of fibre a day. Nutritionists recommend upping that to a full ounce, minimum. Hardly a debilitating change to your daily food consumption. The benefits from such a change are, however, considerable. A large part of the reason why 40 per cent of Britons are constipated is that they eat too little fibre. Ditto, the reason why 20 per cent suffer from diverticular disease. Africans, who eat up to $4^1/_2$ oz of fibre a day do not suffer from these complaints nearly as much as we do. In Britain the average meal stays about three days in the digestive tract; in Africa, because of the high quantity of fibre, the average meal lasts only half a day.

Increasing your fibre intake is simple, and you've already begun the process during the last four weeks. All vegetables and fruit contain dietary fibre to some degree. The skins of fruit and vegetables are full of fibre. Avocados also have a lot. Lettuce isn't exactly brimming with it, but spinach has got a fair portion. Peas and sweetcorn (both of which you can eat pleasantly either raw or cooked, in or out of a salad) broad beans, baked beans (adding a bit of fresh grated ginger reduces flatulence), wholewheat bread, wholewheat pasta, baked potatoes, brown rice and sprouts are all good sources of the stuff, too.

The simplest way to bump up the amount of fibre you eat is to have a bowl of high-fibre cereal such as All-Bran every day, but it is not the best way. There is some evidence that too high a dose of fibre in one go may deprive the body of certain minerals, and it is therefore better to try to get what you need by eating more of fruits and vegetables instead.

So, for these two weeks, make sure you begin eating a plentiful supply of fibre. You can tell when you're eating about the right amount by looking behind you when you've been to the lavatory. A diet with a proper amount produces large, soft stools. A diet with too little results in small, hard ones.

Weeks seven and eight: *Cutting down on saturated fats.* The average diet is much too high in fat generally, but it is the saturated type that is the real baddie. Saturated fats are one of the major contributory factors to heart disease, and heart disease is the most common cause of death in Britain and America. They may also cause breast cancer and metabolic disorders and a variety of other unpleasantnesses. Saturated fats are, with the exception of coconut oil and palm oil, of animal origin and in most cases solid: meat fats, butter, cheese, unskimmed milk and cream are all saturated fats. So are products derived from these, including margarines not labelled high in polyunsaturates, cakes, biscuits, pies, etc. Polyunsaturates come from most vegetable oils (save coconut and palm), fish, nuts and seeds, and some beans such as the soya bean.

Now, obviously, I don't advise you give up all the saturates and eat only unsaturates. But it is a very good idea for your health and figure that you look into the matter and cut back on the amount of saturates you use in your diet. Drink semi-skimmed or unskimmed milk instead of full fat. It might taste a bit watery at first, but you soon get used to it. Two tips for cutting back on butter and cheese: keep your butter soft (it spreads easily and tastes more sickly); grate cheese on to your bread instead of cutting chunks. Make sure you buy only the leanest cuts of meat. When possible, instead of cream substitute yoghurt. If you find that transition particularly hard, try switching first to Greek yoghurt, which tastes very creamy. Yoghurt separates if you heat it too much. The way to get round this is to stabilize it before cooking either by beating an egg into the yoghurt, or by mixing in a teaspoon of cornflour or about a dessertspoon of ordinary flour.

It's very easy to enjoy soy sauce instead of butter on vegetables.

These are all simple, comparatively easy measures which will do your health no end of good.

Weeks nine and ten: *Cutting down on the amount of oil used in frying.* In general, it is wise to cut back not just on saturated fats, but on fats and oils in general. This, probably more than anything else, will help you to find your natural weight. You needn't get carried away, but a few measures would be helpful. Try to grill food instead of frying it. And when you do fry, use less oil and tend to vegetable oils instead of butter or lard. You only need a little to do the job, and you can even buy containers that spray the merest film of oil into the pan. Special dry frying pans use circulating hot air to create the fried effect.

Deep-fried foods like fish and chips don't have to be banned, but it's better to eat them only occasionally. Furthermore, chips vary greatly in the amount of oil they soak up. Chips made from reconstituted potatoes (the ones that are all exactly the same thickness and often crinkle-cut) are the most absorbent, chips made from floury potatoes the next most, and waxy potatoes, particularly if cut thick, the least absorbent.

Weeks eleven and twelve: *Cutting down on sugar.* It is only in the last 100 years that sugar has become a significant part of everybody's diet. More than 200 years ago sugar was one of the great luxuries, which only the very rich could afford, and then in small quantities. For everybody else, sweetness came from fruit and vegetables and, occasionally, a little honey. Now, every year, we eat 100 lbs for every member of the population.

Ideally, we should remove sugars from our diet altogether. They provide no valuable nutrition, only calories. (The 2 lbs of sugar eaten, on average, by every man, woman and child in England, every week, is equivalent to 3400 calories, or about a pound of fat). But to take such a drastic step would be very hard, even if we had the will. Much of the sugar we eat does not come from the sugar you might put in coffee or tea or the cakes, biscuits and sweets you eat, but from sugar in soft drinks and added to tinned foods, sauces, sausages, pies, cereals, yoghurt, etc. Virtually all the commercially prepared foods you buy these days have sugar shoved into them somewhere along the line. Look on the ingredients label: sucrose, glucose, glucose syrup, dextrose, dextrose syrup, fructose, fructose syrup, maltose, maltose syrup, invert sugar, caramel, sorbitol and sugar itself are all given separate entries, but they are all sugars, and on most packets and tins you will find at least one, and probably several, of them mentioned.

In order to cut back, you should start taking foods low in sugar. Among cereals, shredded wheat and puffed wheat are examples that are sugar free. Eat them with gradually less sugar and use fruit to provide the sweetness instead. After a while you will become accustomed to the change and no longer desire the amount you previously thought essential. Sugar is addictive, and you can wean yourself off it very successfully.

Also cut back on it in your tea and coffee, gradually aiming to do without it altogether. Packaged fruit juice is often high in sugar, and jams have to be at least 60 per cent sugar by law. Get low-sugar versions of both. But again, check the ingredients. Even if the label says 'no added sugar', this doesn't mean that there isn't plenty there, introduced by way of concentrated sweet apple juice or the like. Try to eat fewer biscuits and cakes. Many so-called health bars are also very high in sugar. The average fizzy drink contains about ten teaspoonfuls of sugar. Most tins, sauces and pickles are brimming with unnecessary sugar, so, again, go for the low-sugar varieties, or make your own. By cutting back gradually you'll soon lose your taste for the excessive sweetness of the average British diet.

Keep It Up!

Now you've made the most important changes for healthy eating, you'll find that after the three months are up you won't want to go back to your old ways. You may not be perfect yet, but you'll be astonished at how your tastes have changed. You can continue to build on this good basis until your halo shines!

Increasingly, articles are appearing in newspapers and magazines about people who have finally managed to break out of the dieting trap, adopt a healthy lower fat and sugar, higher fibre diet, and found that for the first time ever their bodies have begun to behave as they ought to behave. They have lost weight and arrived at a stable, comfortable level that suits them best. Combined with even a slight exercise programme, these effects are much more forthcoming. Above all, you will be healthier, more energetic and, at last, in control of your body and not in the control of the multi-billion-pound dieting industry.

To your good health!

17

Send These Letters!

There are three letters to cut out and send off: one to your MP, one to a clothes shop of your choice, and one to a magazine. All you have to do is sign, add anything extra you feel like, cut out and post. If you can persuade family and friends – male and female – to add their names, it will become a petition. Better still, make photocopies and send the letters to several MPs, shops and magazines.

SEND TO YOUR MEMBER OF PARLIAMENT

Dear

I ask you to read the following because it concerns issues that are of vital interest to your female constituents.

The issues are dieting and eating disorders.

The incidence of anorexia and bulimia is increasing exponentially. These days children as young as nine are being treated in eating disorder clinics. It is estimated that at least 50 per cent of women suffer from sub-clinical eating disorders.

The current obsession with dieting depends largely on two factors: fashion, and a misconception about weight and health.

1) **Fashion.** The fashion world's obsessive promotion of extreme skinniness obviously influences its audience. This is no longer an unquantifiable connection: an American study found that just as eating disorders are ten and a half times more common among women than men, so advertisements and articles promoting slimming or shape change are ten and a half times more common in women's magazines than in men's.

2) **Weight and health.** It is now known that:

Weight does *not* lower life expectancy. It protects against such conditions as cancer, lung diseases, infertility, complicated pregnancy, osteoporosis. Only extreme degrees of obesity carry health hazards. 'The lastest studies on mortality,' write Drs Wooley and Wooley in the *International Journal of Eating Disorders*, 'show that heavy people are as, or more, healthy than thin people.'

The world's largest ever epidemiological study, completed in 1984 in Norway, involving 1.8 million people, completely confirms this. The highest death and morbidity rates are found among the unfit and underweight. The lowest, among the fit and plump.

Please support the campaign for our nation's health by making sure the government is kept informed of the true facts about health and weight and the evil effects of dieting.

Yours sincerely,

SEND TO A WOMEN'S MAGAZINE

Dear

This letter is an appeal to you to help change the tide of suffering that is overwhelming women and children.

The recent exponential rise in anorexia, bulimia and sub-clinical eating disorders can be directly linked to the pressures of the media. An American study has shown that just as anorexia is ten and a half times more common among women than men, so advertisements and articles promoting slimming or shape change are ten and a half times more common in women's magazines than in men's.

Another survey revealed that magazine models are up to 19 per cent below the weight they should be. Yet being more than 15 per cent below your recommended weight is one of the main diagnostic criteria for anorexia. Is it any wonder that up to half of all women are thought to suffer from disordered eating and that children as young as nine are developing anorexia?

You and your magazine are in a marvellous position to help change this tragic situation.

Weight is not bad for you. It protects against such conditions as cancer, lung diseases, infertility, complicated pregnancy, osteoporosis. Only extreme degrees of obesity carry health hazards. Indeed, Drs Wooley and Wooley report in the *International Journal of Eating Disorders* that 'the latest study on mortality . . . show that heavy people are as, or more, healthy than thin people'.

So, next time you run an article on fitness, health or fashion, please! include normal-sized beauties for illustration. Almost half of British women are size 16 or over. Let your magazine reflect this. You will not only be doing something positive for all women and children, you will also be earning the respect and loyalty of millions of potential readers.

Yours sincerely,

SEND TO A WOMEN'S CLOTHES SHOP

Dear

I have bought clothes at your shop before, and I would do so more often if you catered for a wider range of figures. Please remember that not only are 47 per cent of women size 16+, but that these days it is usual for women to lose or gain significant amounts of weight. Your size 14 customer today might be a size 16 or 18 in a few months, and would have to take her custom elsewhere!

There are three possible changes you could make to your shop which would greatly encourage new customers:

a) Stock a wide variety of clothes for women of all sizes and don't be disrespectful to half your potential customers by hiding your examples of size 16+ clothes at the dim end of the rail and shelf.

b) Do not always use borderline anorexic mannequins. Few average-sized and larger women are fooled into thinking that they, too, will look good in such fashions. Over and over again women have stated that the biggest incentive to purchase is seeing that the clothes look good on someone their own size.

c) Put pressure on your suppliers to create fashions that fit – and suit – women of all sizes. You know it makes good financial sense; make sure they know it too.

By adopting these changes you will not only be tapping into an extremely profitable new market, but will also earn the gratitude of all of us who pass your window.

I look forward to seeing the new alterations in your shop!

Yours sincerely,

SELECT BIBLIOGRAPHY

I have made use of several hundred books and journals during research for this book, and to list them all would swamp the reader with footnotes and bibliographic detail. This list therefore contains only those publications which I found the most helpful and would recommend to readers who want to continue with their own research into the subject. It still looks like a lot, but then it is a very big and often controversial subject. I have added a few of my own comments in a number of places. If there are any further queries, please write to me via the publisher.

I've grouped the sources according to the part of the book for which they were used.

Part One: First, Choose Your Figure

Anderson, A. E., and L. DiDomenico, 'Diet vs. Shape Content of Popular Male and Female Magazines: A Dose-Response Relationship to the Incidence of Eating Disorders?', *International Journal of Eating Disorders*, Vol. 11, No. 3, 1992.

Anderson, J. L., et al., 'Was the Duchess of Windsor Right? A Cross-Cultural Review of the Socioecology of Ideals of Female Body Shape' in *Ethology and Sociobiology*, Vol. 13, (1992)

Anon, *The Art of Beauty* by a Toilet Specialist, The Isobel Handbooks, No. 7. A delightful book published at the turn of the century.

Atkins, J., *Sex in Literature*, Vol. 1 (Calder and Boyars, 1970). Invaluable source book for the subject. This is the first of four volumes, and the best.

Barrett-Connor, E. L., 'Obesity, Atherosclerosis, and Coronary Artery Disease' in *Annals of Internal Medicine*, Vol. 103, No. 6, Pt. 2 (1985).

Bates, G. W., 'Body Weight Control Practice as a Cause of Infertility' in *Clinical Obstetrics and Gynecology*, Vol. 28, No. 3 (September 1985).

Benn, R. T., 'Some Mathematical Properties of Weight-For-Height Indices Used as Parameters of Obesity' in *British Journal of Preventative and Social Medicine*, Vol. 25, 1971.

Bovey, S., *Being Fat Is Not a Sin* (Pandora, 1989). A very intelligent, opinionated, humorous book with an awful title. I recommend it, whatever your shape.

Bradley, P. J., 'Is Obesity an Adventageous Adaptation?' in *International Journal of Obesity*, Vol. 6 (1982).

Bray, G. A., 'Obesity: Historical Developments of Scientific and Cultural Ideas' in *International Journal of Obesity*, Vol. 14 (1990).

Brown, P. J., 'The Biocultural Evolution of Obesity: An Anthropological View', in Per Björntorp and B. N. Brodoff (eds), *Obesity* (J. B. Lippincott Company, 1992).

Caro, T. M., and D. W. Sellen, 'The Reproductive Advantages of Fat in Women' in *Ethology and Sociobiology*, Vol. 11 (1990).

Christensen, L., 'Effects of Eating Behaviour on Mood: A Review of the Literature' in *International Journal of Eating Disorders*, Vol. 14, No. 2 (1993).

Cox, J., 'The Shape of Slimming' in K. Davies, J. Dickey and T. Stratford (eds), *Out of Focus: Writings on Women and the Media* (The Women's Press, 1987).

Drewnowski, A., and S. M. Garn, 'Concerning the Use of Weight Tables to Categorize Patients With Eating Disorders' in *International Journal of Eating Disorders*, Vol. 6, No. 5 (1987).

Editorial, 'In Praise of Embonpoint', *The Lancet*, i, 491 (1987).

Ernsberger, E., and P. Haskew, 'Health Implications of Obesity: An Alternative View' in *The Journal of Obesity and Weight Regulation*, Vol. 6, No. 2 (Summer 1987). A long, brilliant summary of the evidence that obesity is not nearly as dangerous as we've been led to believe. It's hard to get hold of, but well worth the trouble if you're interested.

Flynn, M. A. T., and M. J. Gibney, 'Obesity and Health: Why Slim?', in *Proceedings of the Nutrition Society*, Vol. 50 (1991).

Garner, D. M., and S. C. Wooley, 'Confronting the Failure of Behavioural and Dietary Treatments for Obesity', in *Clinical Psychology Review*, Vol. 11 (1991). Another marvellous survey which I recommend as a starting point (along with Ernsberger and Haskew, above) for anybody interested in a sound, scientific, objective review of the subject.

Harrison, G. G., 'Height–Weight Tables' in *Annals of Internal Medicine*, Vol. 103, No. 6, Pt. 2 (1985). Virtually any one of the articles in this section with 'height–weight' or 'ideal weight' in the title will start you off, pointing out the drawbacks and limited advantages of the weight charts. Together, they give a good insight into the difficulties of apparently simple statistical research and medical accuracy.

Herman, P., and J. Polivy, 'Fat is a Psychological Issue' in *New Scientist*, 16 November 1991.

Hill, A. J., 'Developing Concerns with Dietary Restraint; A Supplement to Tuschl' in *Appetite*, Vol. 14 (1990).

Jarrett, R. J., 'Is There an Ideal Body Weight?' in *British Medical Journal*, Vol. 293 (August 1986).

Jebb, S. A., 'Effect of Weight Cycling Caused by Intermittent Dieting on Metabolic Rate and Body Composition in Obese Women' in *International Journal of Obesity*, Vol. 15 (1991).

Kano, S., *Never Diet Again* (Thorsons Publishing Group, 1990).

Klesges, R. C., T. R. Isbell and L. M. Klesges, 'Relationship Between Dietary Restraint, Energy Intake, Physical Activity, and Body Weight: A Prospective Analysis' in *Journal of Abnormal Psychology*, Vol. 101, No. 4 (1992).

Knapp, T. R., 'A Methodological Critique of the "Ideal Weight" Concept' in *Journal of the American Medical Association*, Vol. 250, No. 4 (1983).

Laessle, R. G., et al., 'Behavioural and Biological Correlates of Dietary Restraint in Normal Life', in *Appetite*, Vol. 12 (1989).

Leader, A., 'The Association of Slimming With Eating Disorders' in *Proceedings of the Nutrition Society*, Vol. 50 (1991). I loved this article. Despite the woefully unpromising title, it is a piece of lovely, humorous writing.

Leys, A., 'Overweight, Obesity, Coronary Heart Disease and Mortality' in *Nutrition Reviews*, Vol. 38, No. 9 (1980).

Lew, E. A., 'Actuarial Contributions to Life Table Analysis', in *National Cancer Institute Monograph*, No. 67 (1985). A useful history of the development of weight table article by the beleaguered head of the Metropolitan Life Insurance Company, which produced the famous tables of 1959 and 1983.

Lowe, M. R., 'Staying on Versus Going Off a Diet: Effects on Eating in Normal Weight and Overweight Individuals' in *International Journal of Eating Disorders*, Vol. 12, No. 4 (1992).

Mahan, L. K., and M. T. Arlin, *Krause's Food, Nutrition and Diet Therapy*, 8th edition (Saunders, Philadelphia 1992). There is a variety of nutrition textbooks about, I found this one the best.

Mann, G. V., 'Obesity, The Nutritional Spook' in *American Journal of Public Health*, Vol. 61, No. 8 (1971).

Mann, G. V., 'The Influence of Obesity on Health' in *New England Journal of Medicine*, 25 July 1974.

McCluskey, S. E., 'Dietary Restraint – A Useful Concept?' in *Appetite*, Vol. 14 (1990).

Morris, A., T. Cooper and P. J. Cooper, 'The Changing Shape of Female Fashion Models', in *International Journal of Eating Disorders*, Vol. 8, No. 5 (1989).

National Institutes of Health Consensus Development Conference Statement, 'Health Implication of Obesity' in *Annals of Internal Medicine*, Vol. 103, No. 6, Pt. 2 (1985).

Ogden, J., *Fat Chance!* (Routledge, 1992). A good introduction to the anti-slimming evidence, but, infuriatingly, without a bibliography or any other form of reference section.

Ogden, J., and L. Greville, 'Cognitive Changes to Preloading in Restrained and Unrestrained Eaters as Measured by the Stroop Task' in *International Journal of Eating Disorders*, Vol. 14, No. 2 (1993).

Parish, P., *Medicines: A Guide for Everybody*, 6th edition (Penguin, 1987). These were splendid editions, particularly useful in Britain since our doctors are world famous for their reluctance to give out proper information about the drugs they prescribe. I've not come across a later edition (they used to come out every few years or so).

Perri, M. G., A. M. Nezu and B. J. Viegener, *Improving the Long-Term Management of Obesity* (John Wiley and Sons, 1992).

Prentice, A. M., et al., 'Physiological Responses to Slimming' in *Proceedings of the Nutrition Society*, Vol. 50 (1991).

Pyle, R. L., et al., 'The Use of Weight Tables to Categorize Patients with Eating Disorders' in *International Journal of Eating Disorders*, Vol. 5, No. 2 (1986).

Richardson, S. A., et al., 'Cultural Uniformity in Reaction to Physical Disabilities', in *American Sociological Review*, Vol. 26 (1961).

Rodin, J., et al., 'Weight Cycling and Fat Distribution' in *International Journal of Obesity*, Vol. 14 (1990).

Rodin, J., 'Psychological and Behavioural Determinants of Regional Fat Deposition' in G. Ailhaud et al. (eds) *Obesity in Europe 91* (John Libbey, 1992).

Rogers, P. J., et al., 'Nutritional Influences on Mood and Cognitive Performance: The Menstrual Cycle, Caffeine and Dieting' in *Proceedings of the Nutrition Society*, Vol. 51 (1992).

Rogers, P. J., and M. W. Green, 'Dieting, Dietary Restraint and Cognitive Performance' in *British Journal of Clinical Psychology*, Vol. 32 (1993).

Sanders, T., quoted in H. Nowicka, 'We're Happy to be the Fat of the Land', *Independent on Sunday*, 21 November 1993

Sanders, T., and P. Bazalgette, *You Don't Have to Diet!* (Bantam Press, 1994). Plenty of good information, carefully presented. Dr Sanders, a nutritionist at King's College, London, has made a name for himself as a straightforward, responsible, popular detailer of dietary facts. Rather an oddity, in other words.

Sichieri, R., J. E. Everhart and V. S. Hubbard, 'Relative Weight Classifications in the Assessment of Underweight and Overweight in the United States' in *International Journal of Obesity*, Vol. 16 (1992).

Silverstein, B., B. Peterson and L. Perdue, 'Some Correlates of Bodily Attractiveness for Women', in *International Journal of Eating Disorders*, Vol. 5, No. 5 (1986).

Silverstein, B., et al., 'Possible Causes of the Thin Standard of Bodily Attractiveness for Women', in *International Journal of Eating Disorders*, Vol. 5, No. 5 (1986).

Stini, W., 'Body Composition and Longevity: Is There a Longevous Morphotype?' in *Medical Anthropology*, Vol. 13 (1991).

Tarui, S., et al., 'Visceral Fat Obesity: Anthropological and Pathophysiological Aspects' in *International Journal of Obesity*, Vol. 15 (1991).

Tokunaga, K., et al., 'Ideal Body Weight Estimated From the Body Mass Index With the Lowest Morbidity' in *International Journal of Obesity*, Vol. 15 (1991).

Treasure, J., 'Comments on Some Theoretical Considerations: Dietary Restraint to Binge Eating' in *Appetite*, Vol. 14 (1990).

Tuschl, R. J., 'From Dietary Restraint to Binge Eating: Some Theoretical Considerations' in *Appetite*, Vol. 14 (1990)

Vague, J., et al., 'Android and Gynoid Obesities, Past and Present' in J. Vague et al. (eds) *Metabolic Complications of Human Obesities* (Excerpta Medica, 1985).

Wardle, J., 'Compulsive Eating and Dietary Restraint' in *British Journal of Clinical Psychology*, Vol. 26 (1987).

Wardle, J., 'Overeating: A Regulatory Behaviour in Restrained Eaters' in *Appetite*, Vol. 14 (1990).

Wiseman, C. V., et al., 'Cultural Expectations of Thinness in Women: An Update', in *International Journal of Eating Disorders*, Vol. 11, No. 1 (1992).

Part Two: What are the Options for Losing Weight?

Achenbach, T. M., and C. T. Howell, 'Are American Children's Problems Getting Worse: A 13-Year Comparison', in *Journal of the American Academy of Child and Adolescent Psychiatry*, Vol. 32, No. 6 (1993).

Buist, J. S., 'Mr Banting's "Excellent Adviser" ' in *The Practitioner*, Vol. 194 (March 1965). A pleasant piece. Banting's adviser was a Dr Harvey. Also a good indication of how times have changed. The diet was mild, the weight loss gentle; Banting was self-effacing, and Dr Harvey modest.

Casper, R. C., and D. Offer, 'Weight and Dieting Concerns in Adolescents, Fashion or Symptom?' in *Pediatrics*, Vol. 86, No. 3 (1990).

Deitz, W. H., and R. Hartung, 'Changes in Height Velocity of Obese Preadolescents During Weight Reduction', in *American Journal of Diseases of Children*, Vol. 139 (1985).

Fichter, M. M., 'The Anorexia Nervosa of Franz Kafka', in *International Journal of Eating Disorders*, Vol. 6, No. 3 (1987).

Field, A. E., et al., 'The Relationship of Caloric Intake to Frequency of Dieting Among Preadolescent and Adolescent Girls', in *Journal of the American Academy of Child and Adolescent Psychiatry*, Vol. 32, No. 6 (1993).

Freedman, R., *Beauty Bound* (Columbus Books, 1988).

Fried, R., and W. Vandereycken, 'The Peter Pan Syndrome; was James M. Barrie Anorexic?', in *International Journal of Eating Disorders*, Vol. 8, No. 3 (1989).

Friedman, R. B., 'Fad Diets; Evaluation of Five Common Types' in *Postgraduate Medicine*, Vol. 79, No. 1 (1986).

Garrow, J. S., 'Morbid Obesity: Medical or Surgical Treatment? The Case for Medical Treatment' in *International Journal of Obesity*, Vol. 11, Suppl. 3 (1987).

Hamilton, J. W., 'Gastric Balloons to Treat Obesity' in *Postgraduate Medicine*, Vol. 83, No. 6 (1988).

Hill, A. J., 'Causes and Consequences of Dieting and Anorexia' in *Proceedings of the Nutrition Society*, Vol. 52 (1993).

Hill, A. J., 'Pre-adolescent Dieting: Implications for Eating Disorders', *International Review of Psychiatry*, Vol. 5 (1993).

Hill, A. J., S. Oliver and P. J. Rogers, 'Eating in the Adult World: The Rise of Dieting in Childhood and Adolescence', in *British Journal of Clinical Psychology*, Vol. 31 (1992).

Hsu, L. K. G., 'The Gender Gap in Eating Disorders: Why are the Eating Disorders More Common Among Women?', in *Clinical Psychology Review*, Vol. 9 (1989).

Howard, A. N., 'The Historical Development, Efficacy and Safety of Very-Low-Calorie Diets' in *International Journal of Obesity*, Vol. 5 (1981).

Jung, R. T., *A Colour Atlas of Obesity* (Wolfe Medical Publications Ltd, 1990).

Killen, J. D., et al., 'Is Puberty a Risk Factor for Eating Disorders?' in *American Journal of Diseases of Children*, Vol. 146 (1992).

Kreipe, R. E., and G. B. Forbes, 'Osteoporosis: A "New Morbidity" for

Dieting Female Adolescents?', in *Pediatrics*, Vol. 86, No. 3 (1990).

Lifshitz, F., and N. Moses, 'Growth Failure: A Complication of Dietary Treatment of Hypercholesterolemia' in *American Journal of Diseases of Children*, Vol. 143 (1989).

Løvig, T., et al., 'Gastric Banding for Morbid Obesity: Five Years Follow-Up' in *International Journal of Obesity*, Vol. 17 (1993).

Low, B. S., 'Fat and Deception' in *Ethnology and Sociobiology*, Vol. 11 (1990).

Maloney, M. J., et al., 'Dieting Behaviour and Eating Attitudes in Children', in *Pediatrics*, Vol. 84, No. 3 (1989).

Mogadam, M., 'Nutritional Fads' in *The American Journal of Gastroenterology*, Vol. 85, No. 3 (1990).

Orbach, S., *Fat Is a Feminist Issue* (Arrow, 1986). (First British edition, (1978.) The classic in the field, and though I have reservations about it (see Chapter 9), it is still an important and provocative book.

Parry-Jones, B., and W. Ll. Parry-Jones, 'Bulimia: An Archival Review of Its History in Psychosomatic Medicine', in *International Journal of Eating Disorders*, Vol. 10, No. 2 (1991).

Pasquali, R., et al., 'Mechanisms of Action of the Intragastric Balloon in Obesity: Effects on Hunger and Satiety' in *Appetite*, Vol. 15 (1990).

Pate, J. E., et al., 'Cross-Cultural Patterns in Eating Disorders: A Review', in *Journal of the American Academy of Child and Adolescent Psychiatry*, Vol. 31, No. 5 (1992).

Paterson, *The A for Allergy Diet Book* (Pathway, 1986).

Sanders, T. A. B., R. Woolfe and E. Rantzen, 'Controlled Evaluation of Slimming Diets: Use of Television for Recruitment' in *The Lancet*, Vol. 336 (1990). Esther Rantzen's transformation from telly star to co-author of a paper appearing in Britain's premier scientific journal.

Schwartz, H., *Never Satisfied: A Cultural History of Diets, Fantasies and Fat* (The Free Press, 1986). Full of curious information written in a maddening, pompous style.

Shute, J., *Life-Size* (Mandarin, 1993). Harsh novel about anorexia.

Trimmer, E., *The Complete Book of Slimming and Diets* (Piatkus, 1981). Lots of now rather old-fashioned information.

Wardle, J., and S. Beales, 'Restraint, Body Image and Food Attitudes in Children from 12 to 18 Years', in *Appetite*, Vol. 7 (1986).

Wolf, A., et al., 'Activity, Inactivity, and Obesity: Racial, Ethnic, and Age Differences Among Schoolgirls', in *American Journal of Public Health*, Vol. 83, No. 11 (1993).

Wolf, N., *The Beauty Myth* (Vintage, 1990). I have mixed feelings about this book. It is strong, angry, energetic, but it's a good idea to check up on her facts. In a number of places emotive argument takes precedence over good research, and she can be a bit wild with her statistics.

Wooley, O. W., and S. Wooley, 'The Beverly Hills Eating Disorder: the Mass Marketing of Anorexia Nervosa' in *International Journal of Eating Disorders*, Vol. 1, No. 3 (1982).

Yates, A., 'Current Perspectives on the Eating Disorders: I. History, Psychological and Biological Aspects', in *Journal of the American Academy of Child and Adolescent Psychology*, Vol. 28 (1989).

Young, E. A., 'United Sciences of America, Incorporated: An "Optimal" Diet' in *Annals of Internal Medicine*, Vol. 107 (1987).

Part Three: What Really Works?

Sanders, T., *The Food Revolution* (Bantam, 1991). This doesn't tell you what really works, but it gives an extraordinarily detailed account of our eating habits and what's wrong with them.